Neuroscience for Pre-Clinical Students

Neuroscience for Pre-Clinical Students

RENÉE J. LECLAIR

PDF AND EPUB FREE ONLINE AT: HTTPS://DOI.ORG/10.21061/NEUROSCIENCE

VIRGINIA TECH CARILION SCHOOL OF MEDICINE IN ASSOCIATION WITH VIRGINIA TECH PUBLISHING
BLACKSBURG, VA

Suggested citation: LeClair, Renée (2022). *Neuroscience for Pre-Clinical Students*. Roanoke: Virginia Tech Carilion School of Medicine. https://doi.org/10.21061/neuroscience. Licensed with CC BY-NC-SA 4.0 https://creativecommons.org/licenses/by-nc-sa/4.0.

Publisher: This work is published by the Virginia Tech Carilion School of Medicine in association with Virginia Tech Publishing, a division of the University Libraries at Virginia Tech.

Virginia Tech Carilion School of Medicine 2 Riverside Circle Roanoke, VA 24016 USA

Virginia Tech Publishing University Libraries at Virginia Tech 560 Drillfield Drive Blacksburg, VA 24061 USA https://publishing.vt.edu publishing@vt.edu

This work is also distributed by LibreTexts, Davis, CA USA info@libretexts.org. Note: The LibreTexts version of this work at https://med.libretexts.org/@go/page/35685 may differ from this version.

Peer review: This book has undergone single-blind peer review by five external reviewers.

Accessibility statement: Virginia Tech Publishing is committed to making its publications accessible in accordance with the Americans with Disabilities Act of 1990. The Pressbooks (HTML) and ePub versions of this text are tagged structurally and include alternative text, which allows for machine readability.

Publication cataloging information:
LeClair, Renée, author
Neuroscience for Pre-Clinical Students / Renée LeClair

ISBN 978-1-949373-80-6 (PDF)
ISBN 978-1-949373-81-3 (ePub)
ISBN 978-1-949373-82-0 (Pressbooks) https://pressbooks.lib.vt.edu/neuroscience
ISBN 978-1-949373-84-4 (Print)
URI (Universal Resource Identifier) http://hdl.handle.net/10919/105408
DOI https://doi.org/10.21061/neuroscience

1. Neurochemistry -- Textbooks
   Title QP356.3 $b .L43

Disclaimer: The information in this textbook is intended for educational purposes only and is not meant to take the place of medical care, diagnoses, or services. Please see your healthcare provider about any health concerns.

Cover art: Brain by Mahmure Alp from The Noun Project. CC BY.
Illustration and cover design: Kindred Grey

Contents

Introduction

Neuroscience for Pre-Clinical Students is designed to fill a gap in undergraduate medical education (UME) and support preclerkship education in the content area of biochemical neuroscience. Its content is aligned to USMLE(r) (United States Medical Licensing Examination) providing coverage of topics including: neuroenergetics, neurotransmitters, neuropeptides, and amino acid metabolism and heritable disorders of degradation. Unlike traditional textbooks, the organization of this resource is driven by curricular structure, rather than subject area. As the format and design of UME differs across many programs, this resource is purposefully brief and flexible, allowing for rapid adaptation across programs. The resource is organized into small chapters that can be used to support student preparation in any arrangement. The sections are not intended to be all-inclusive, but rather primers for applied content delivery. Similarly, clinical context is only briefly discussed allowing the user to apply the basic content (delivered here) in the clinical context used by their specific curricular structure. In our curriculum, these topic areas are interwoven into problem-based learning cases. The cases and clinical correlates change regularly and having the flexibility of these short resources that can be applied to many scenarios across the first and second years of our curriculum is beneficial.

Over the past twenty years, medical education has undergone a rapid curricular restructuring. This is in part due to recommendations of the Flexner report,[1] coupled with the changes observed in millennial[2] and iGen learners. To accommodate the integration of additional core competencies, the majority of medical programs have moved away from discipline-based delivery and currently use some form of integrated curricular format.[3] This allows material to be presented in a more clinically realistic and pertinent format without the constraints of artificial discipline silos. This movement has had positive impacts on programmatic outcomes and student performance, but it has presented some challenges for curricular design, student engagement and educational resources.

The creation of this resource was intended to address three predominant challenges in medical education: need, student engagement and cost of textbooks. Although contemporary medical curricula have moved to a cohesive, integrated format, the required textbooks for undergraduate medical education remain traditional and discipline-based. In the absence of an integrated resource, students are requested to purchase and juggle preparation materials between many different discipline-based textbooks. Traditional textbooks are often designed to support subject-based courses, rather than a clinically centered education. (Medical schools are educating future physicians, not future biochemists, physiologists, etc.) A high volume of content, some of it lacking alignment with class sessions coupled with restrictions on student contact time imposed by accrediting bodies, means that faculty across the country are having to rethink preparation materials to facilitate efficient, focused learning experiences.

This resource is intended to provide learners with a high-level view of relevant topical areas that will be further elaborated on within the classroom setting. Unlike other traditional textbooks, it is not intended to include all content a learner would need about the relevant subject area but to function as a stepping stone towards mastery of the content.

As programs embrace the philosophy of student-directed learning embedded in adult learning theory, more simplified readily available resources will be essential to support this fast-paced learning of health professional educational programs. The short-divided nature of the resource makes it flexible and adaptable to many different curricular settings as topic areas can be quickly divided or separated for ideal use. While there are many factors that can contribute to a student's lack of preparation, lengthy textbook resources for a single integrated classroom session have a significant negative impact. So while an integrated curricular model enhances many aspects of learning, it makes using traditional textbooks cumbersome and disjointed for students. This resource hopes to address this concern.

Finally, there is a wealth of "medical" content freely accessible online, and students can find themselves spending a significant amount of time trying to identify alternative resources that may—or may not—be appropriate. Faculty taking ownership to identify and adapt realistic materials for each session reduces the concern that students are finding misinformation through internet sources, and this project allows faculty to create a resource that harnesses the best attributes of many different formats into a product that best supports the learning environment. Otherwise, external online resources are also likely to contain extraneous content that is not aligned with the classroom learning objectives (akin to subject-based textbook chapters), so it can also reduce the perceived worth of preparation. If the integrated resource is generated correctly, concisely and accurately by the faculty, the students will gain trust, rely on the vetted resources and prepare for the active classroom.

— Renée LeClair

Notes

1. Cooke M, Irby DM, Ph D, et al. American Medical Education 100 Years after the Flexner Report. 2006:1339-1344.
2. Roberts DH, Newman LR, Schwartzstein RM. Twelve tips for facilitating Millennials' learning. Medical Teacher. 2012;34:274-278.
3. VanTassel-Baska J, Wood S. The integrated curriculum model (ICM). Learning and Individual Differences. 2010;20(4):345-357.

Acknowledgments

Funding and In-Kind Support

Publication of this work is made possible in part through the support of VIVA (Virtual Library of Virginia), LibreTexts, the Open Education Initiative of the University Libraries at Virginia Tech, and Virginia Tech Publishing.

Peer Reviewers

Lauren Kennedy-Metz, Instructor of Surgery, Harvard Medical School
Kristofer Rau, Assistant Professor of Basic Science Education, Virginia Tech Carilion School of Medicine

Editorial Team

Managing Editor: Anita Walz
Graphic Design and Editorial Assistance: Kindred Grey
Alternative Text: Sophia DeSimone

Special Thanks

Henry Jakubowski, Emeritus, College of Saint Benedict and Saint John's University
Delmar Larson, Founder, LibreTexts
Christa Miller, Accessible Technologies, Virginia Tech

About the Author

Renée J. LeClair is an Associate Professor in the Department of Basic Science Education at the Virginia Tech Carilion School of Medicine, where her role is to engage activities that support the departmental mission of developing an integrated medical experience using evidence-based delivery grounded in the science of learning. She received a Ph.D. at Rice University and completed a postdoctoral fellowship at the Maine Medical Center Research Institute in vascular biology. She became involved in medical education, curricular renovation, and implementation of innovative teaching methods during her first faculty appointment, at the University of New England, College of Osteopathic Medicine. In 2013, she moved to a new medical school, University of South Carolina, School of Medicine, Greenville. The opportunities afforded by joining a new program and serving as the Chair of the Curriculum committee provided a blank slate for creative curricular development and close involvement with the accreditation process. During her tenure she developed and directed a team-taught student-centered undergraduate medical course that integrated the scientific and clinical sciences to assess all six-core competencies of medical education.

Instructor Resources

How to Adopt This Book

Instructors reviewing, adopting, or adapting this textbook are encouraged to register at https://bit.ly/interest-preclinical. This assists Virginia Tech's Open Education Initiative in assessing the impact of the book and allows us to more easily alert instructors of additional resources, features and opportunities.

Finding Additional Resources for Your Course

The main landing page for the book is http://hdl.handle.net/10919/105408.

This page includes:

- Links to multiple electronic versions of the textbook (PDF, ePub, HTML)
- Links to the instructor resource-sharing portal
- Link to errata document https://pressbooks.lib.vt.edu/neuroscience
- Links to other books within this series

Sharing Resources You've Created

Have you created any supplementary materials for use with Neuroscience for Pre-Clinical Students such as presentation slides, activities, test items, or a question bank? If so, please consider sharing your materials related to this open textbook. Please tell us about resources you wish to share by using this form: https://bit.ly/interest-preclinical or by directly sharing resources under an open license to the public-facing instructor sharing portal https://www.oercommons.org/groups/pre-clinical-resources/10133.

Customizing This Book

The Creative Commons Attribution NonCommercial-ShareAlike 4.0 license https://creativecommons.org/licenses/by-nc-sa/4.0/legalcode on this book allows customization and redistribution which is NonCommercial, that is "not primarily intended for or directed towards commercial advantage or monetary compensation."

Best practices for attribution are provided at https://wiki.creativecommons.org/wiki/ Best_practices_for_attribution.

This book is hosted in PDF and ePub in VTechWorks, in HTML in Pressbooks and via the LibreTexts platform. Pressbooks and LibreTexts platforms both offer customization/remixing.

Feedback

To report an error or omission, please use https://bit.ly/feedback-preclinical.

We welcome additional feedback at publishing@vt.edu.

1. Neuron and astrocyte metabolism

Learning Objectives

- Describe the metabolic pathway of glucose and its metabolites and how they are utilized in the brain, and list the major energy-consuming processes in the brain.
- Describe the role of glial cells in neuron metabolism.
- Evaluate the interaction between astrocytes and neurons in the regulation of cerebral blood flow.
- Compare the metabolic profile of neurons and astrocytes.
- Review basic metabolic pathways, including: glycolysis, glycogen synthesis/olysis, transaminations, and glutathione synthesis.

The adult brain consumes about 25 percent of the glucose-derived energy and 20 percent of oxygen is dedicated to cerebral functions. The primary fuel to support the high energy demands of this tissue is supplied in the form of glucose, however, not all neuronal tissues oxidize glucose to the same extent. This section will address the distinct metabolic differences between astrocyte and neuronal metabolic profiles and how this interplay is essential for brain metabolic homeostasis.

As a brief review, glucose is taken up by the brain in an insulin-independent manner. The brain oxidizes glucose under most conditions with the exception of starvation states. Once the glucose is phosphorylated to glucose 6-phosphate (by hexokinase), it has three potential fates (figure 1.1):

1. Glycolysis (either leading to lactate production or mitochondrial metabolism),
2. Pentose phosphate pathway (PPP), or
3. Glycogen synthesis (only in astrocytes).

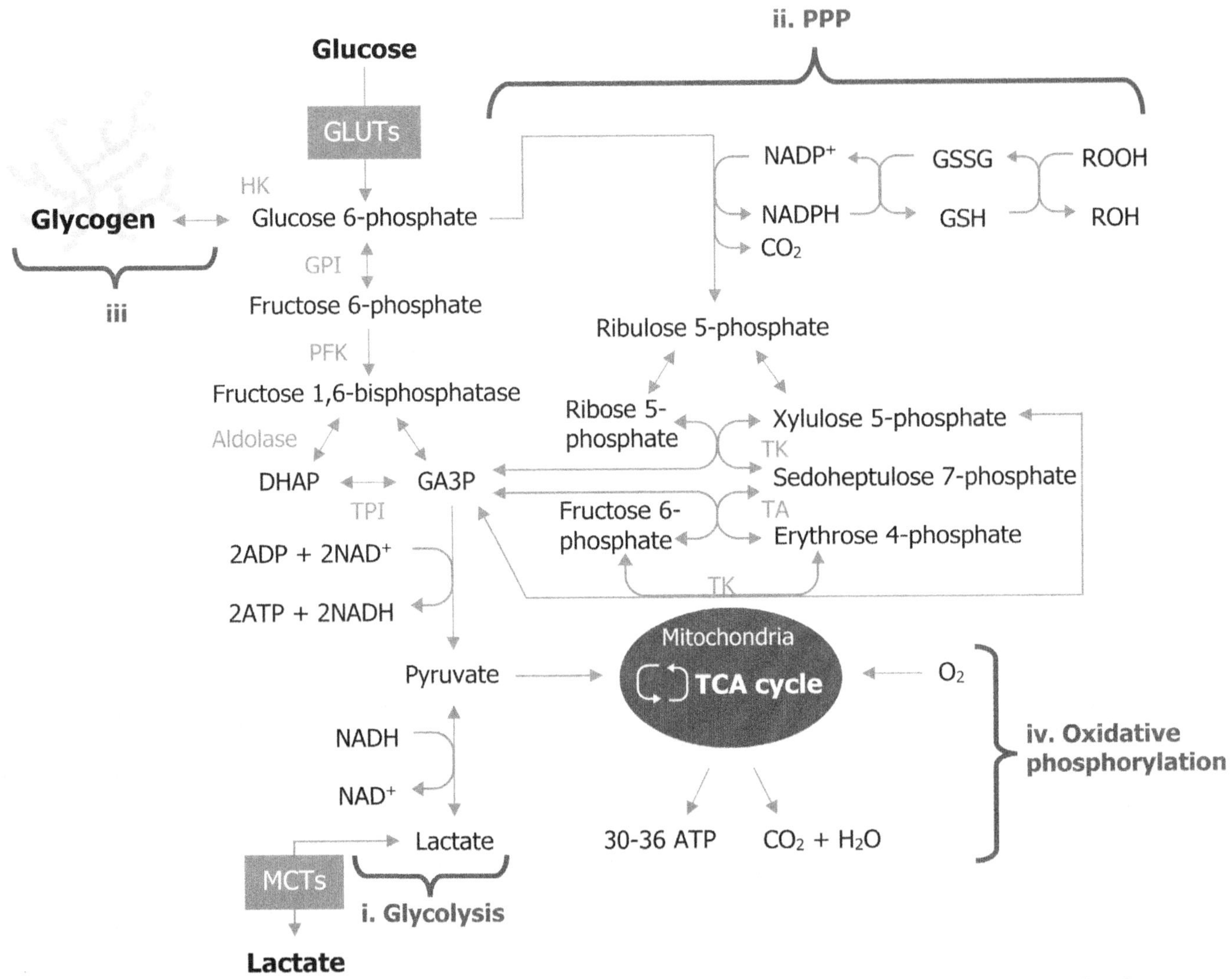

Figure 1.1: Potential fates of glucose oxidation. i. Glucose is oxidized to lactate; ii. Glucose is oxidized through the pentose phosphate pathway (PPP); iii. Glucose is stored as glycogen, which only occurs in astrocytes; iv. Pyruvate can be oxidized through the mitochondria but is not a primary fate. (GLUTs: glucose transporters; MCTs: monocarboxylate transporters; TCA: tricarboxylic acid; DHAP: dihydroxyacetone phosphate; GA3P: glyceraldehyde 3-phosphate)

What is unique to the brain is that not all cell types oxidize glucose to the same extent, but there is a tight coupling that exists between cell types to support both energy demand and glutamate-mediated neurotransmission. This compartmentalized, coupled metabolism between neurons and astrocytes is essential for ATP production, neuronal excitability, and adaptations to stress.

Note

In the context of this chapter, *oxidative metabolism* refers to the oxidation of a substrate (glucose) through mitochondrial metabolism versus *glycolytic metabolism*, which refers to the oxidation of glucose to lactate.

Neuron metabolism

To support the high energy demands imposed on neurons, they sustain a high rate of oxidative metabolism for ATP production compared to astrocytes. Despite this high rate of mitochondrial metabolism, glucose uptake is reduced when compared to astrocytes, in part due to the use of lactate as an energy source. Neurons show a preference for lactate over glucose when both substrates are present. There are several reasons why sustaining a low glycolytic rate but high oxidative rate is preferred in this tissue:

1. The bifunctional enzyme phosphofructokinase 2 (PFK2) is virtually absent in neurons, due to its constant proteasomal degradation. This enzyme is responsible for the generation of fructose 2,6-bisphosphate, which is an allosteric activator of the glycolytic enzyme phosphofructokinase 1 (PFK1).
2. Elevated glycolytic flux impairs metabolism through the PPP. Neurons purposefully reduce glycolytic flux to maintain metabolism through the PPP—which is essential for the production of NADPH through the reaction catalyzed by glucose 6-phosphate dehydrogenase.

To accommodate these two processes, neurons preferentially utilize lactate, which can be readily converted to pyruvate and enter the mitochondria (figure 1.2). The lactate required for neuronal metabolism is produced by astrocytic glucose oxidation and is discussed below.

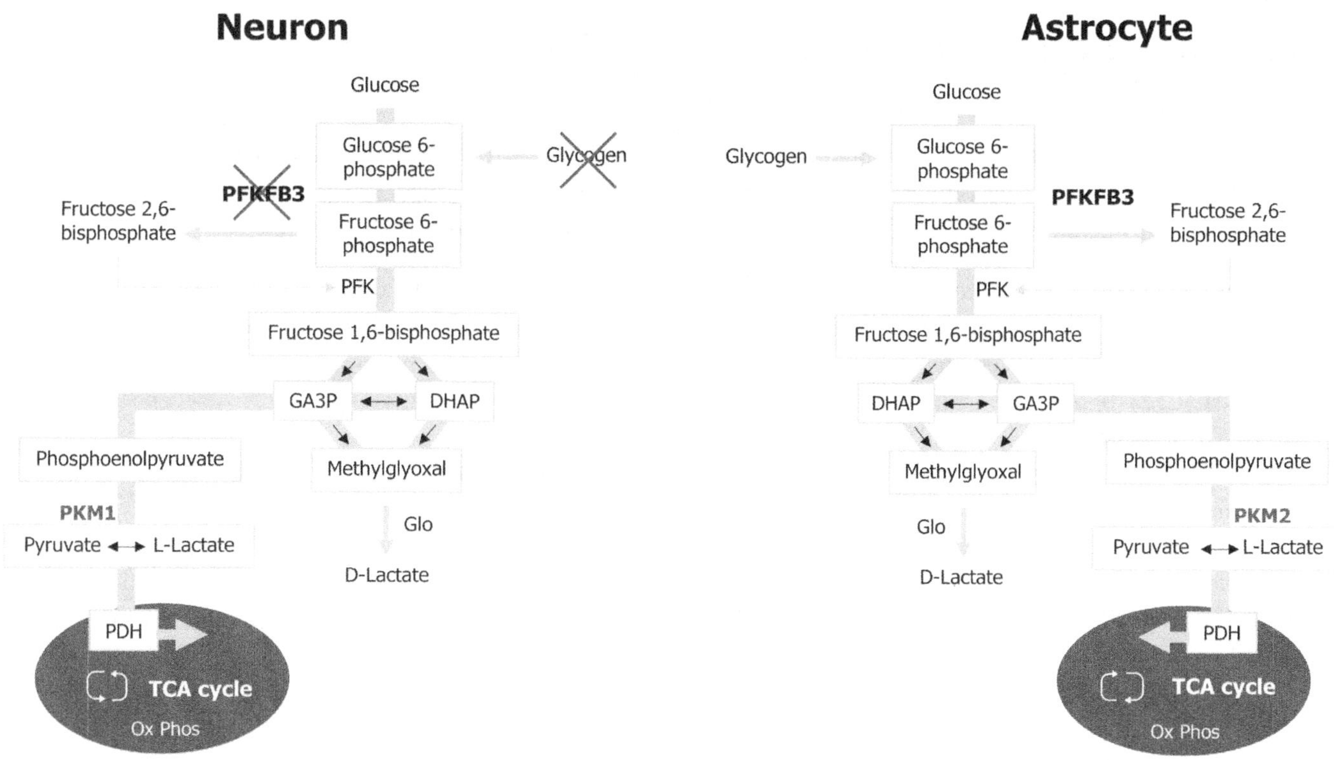

Figure 1.2: Comparison of neuron and astrocyte metabolism. (PDH: pyruvate dehydrogenase complex; PKM1/2: pyruvate kinase isoforms M1 and M2; TCA: tricarboxylic acid; DHAP: dihydroxyacetone phosphate; GA3P: glyceraldehyde 3-phosphate)

Astrocyte metabolism

Within the brain, astrocytes outnumber neurons but have reduced demand for ATP. Although astrocytes display lower oxidative rates when compared to neurons, they have elevated glycolytic rates and avidly take up glucose to support this. Astrocytes primarily metabolize glucose to lactate (rather than through mitochondrial metabolism) and release the lactate in the extracellular space. Astrocytes support this glycolytic profile through the alteration of several key glycolytic enzymes.

1. Astrocytes have increased expression of PFK2, which assists with the elevated glycolytic rate via the allosteric activation of PFK1 by fructose 2,6-bisphosphate.
2. Astrocytes have reduced expression of the aspartate/glutamate carrier (AGC), a component of the malate-aspartate shuttle, which facilitates the transfer of reducing equivalents from the cytosol to the mitochondria. As a result, the conversion of pyruvate to lactate in the cytosol is needed to maintain a high NAD^+/NADH ratio, which is essential to sustain a high glycolytic rate.
3. Finally, the conversion of pyruvate to lactate in astrocytes is also favored by both reduced expression and phosphorylation-mediated inactivation of the pyruvate dehydrogenase complex (figure 1.2).

Astrocyte-mediated neurotransmitter recycling

To terminate synaptic transmission and maintain neuronal excitability, astrocytes play a key role in the rapid removal of neurotransmitters from the synaptic cleft. The removal of glutamate is specifically critical as this is the primary excitatory neurotransmitter, and overstimulation of glutamate receptors is highly toxic to neurons.

Astrocytes recycle glutamate through sodium-dependent high-affinity glutamate transporters. Following glutamate uptake, astrocytes also play an important role in transferring this neurotransmitter back to neurons. This transfer is achieved by a process called the glutamate-glutamine cycle, which involves both glutamine synthetase (GS) and glutaminase (GLS) (figure 1.3).

1. First, glutamate is converted to glutamine by the astrocyte-specific enzyme GS.
2. Glutamine is then transferred to neurons and converted back to glutamate via deamination by GLS.

It is also important to note that astrocytes are the only neural cell type expressing pyruvate carboxylase, a key enzyme in the main anaplerotic pathway in the brain. This allows astrocytes to effectively synthesize glutamate from glucose, making them the cell type responsible for the replenishment of brain glutamate.

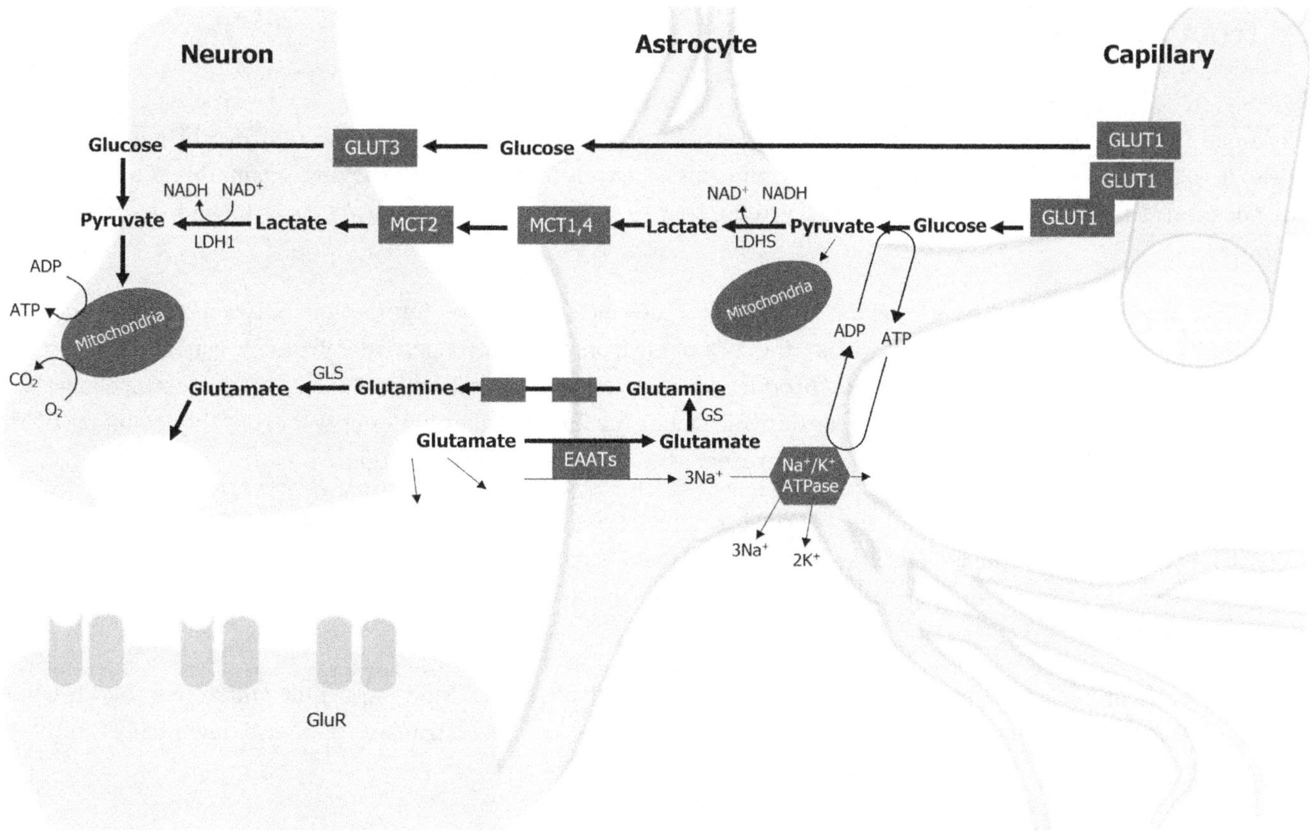

Figure 1.3: Lactate and glutamate shuttling between the astrocyte and the neuron. (GS: glutamine synthetase; GLS: glutaminase; LDH: lactate dehydrogenase; EAATs: excitatory amino acid transporters; MCT: monocarboxylate transporter; GluR: glutamate receptor).

Astrocyte-neuron lactate shuttle

To this point, we have addressed the need for lactate in the neuron to sustain high demands for ATP, astrocyte glycolytic activity and elevated glucose uptake, and the role of the astrocyte in glutamate recycling. These three processes are not unrelated, and the juxtaposition in energy needs and glucose uptake between these two cell types can be reconciled when we address the role of the astrocyte-neuron lactate shuttle (ANLS).

The premise of this shuttle is threefold:

1. Neuronal activity increases extracellular glutamate (via glutamatergic neurotransmission), which is avidly taken up via an Na^+-dependent mechanism.
2. The resulting increase in intracellular Na^+ activates the Na^+/K^+ ATP-ase and increases ATP consumption.
3. The fall of ATP increases lactate production, which is released into the extracellular space.

Finally, lactate can be used as an energy substrate for neurons for oxidative-derived ATP production (figure 1.3).

Astrocyte glycogen stores

Glycogen is the largest energy reserve of the brain and provides a source of glucose that can be rapidly mobilized without ATP. Stores of glycogen in the brain are almost exclusively localized to astrocytes. Again, this observation raises the question as to why the main energy reserve in the brain is found in astrocytes rather than the high-energy-requiring neurons.

Much like the lactate shuttle, glycogen metabolism relies heavily on the interaction between the two cell types to preserve metabolic homeostasis within the brain environment. Glycogen mobilization can support astrocyte metabolism, but it also increases lactate production and the concentration of lactate in the extracellular space. Considering the role of astrocytic glucose-derived lactate in fueling neuronal energy needs, this coupling of these compartmentalized metabolic processes helps preserve the function of each cell type.

Glycogen also has other roles in the normal brain. The amount of glycogen is under dynamic control of neurotransmitters. For example, decreased neuronal activity, such as in sleep, correlates with increased levels of brain glycogen, while an increase in neuronal activity, such as in the awake brain, is associated with a decrease in glycogen levels in active areas.

As a whole, these observations demonstrate that astrocytic glycogen plays an important and active role in complex brain physiological functions, in particular through an astrocyte-to-neuron transfer of energy metabolites in the form of lactate.

The role of astrocyte-neuron interactions to reduce oxidative stress

Oxidative injury is a key feature of several neuropathological conditions such as stroke, traumatic brain injury, and neurodegenerative diseases. There are several factors that contribute to increased brain vulnerability to oxidative stress, including its high rate of oxidative energy metabolism (a process inevitably generating reactive oxygen species (ROS) as a byproduct), its high unsaturated fatty acids content (which are prone to lipid peroxidation), and its relatively low intrinsic antioxidant capacity.

Although neurons have a higher proportion of oxidative metabolism, they have few defenses against oxidative stress. Astrocytes, alternatively, have significant levels of ROS-detoxifying enzymes, including glutathione, heme oxygenase 1, glutathione peroxidase, glutathione S-transferase, catalase, and thioredoxin reductase. As a result, astrocytes are much more resistant to cellular damage by H_2O_2, NO, peroxinitrites, and 6-hydroxydopamine compared to neurons.

Astrocytes also play an important protective role for neurons, suggesting that neurons are dependent on the high antioxidant potential of astrocytes for their own defense against oxidative stress.

One way in which astrocytes provide protection is through the shuttling of glutathione (GSH) precursors from astrocytes to neurons. GSH—the most abundant antioxidant molecule in the brain—either acts directly as a ROS scavenger or can be used as a substrate for glutathione S-transferase or glutathione peroxidase. Both cell types can synthesize the GSH tripeptide, but neurons are highly dependent on astrocytes for the supply of the precursor amino acids necessary for their own GSH synthesis.

The reduction of peroxides catalyzed by glutathione peroxidase generates glutathione disulfide (GSSG, the oxidized form of GSH). GSH can subsequently be regenerated from GSSG by the action of the enzyme glutathione reductase, using NADPH as an electron donor. This process is essential for the maintenance of GSH in its reduced form, and thus for its availability for the detoxification of ROS. As a consequence, constant NADPH supply is essential for the maintenance of the cellular redox state.

NADPH production is mainly achieved by the metabolism of glucose via the PPP, thereby coupling glutathione recycling to glucose utilization. NADPH is more abundant in astrocytes than in neurons, and astrocytes have a higher basal PPP activity rate and a better capacity to stimulate this pathway in response to oxidative stress.

Astrocyte-neuron impact on cerebral blood flow

The metabolic interplay between astrocytes and neurons goes beyond substrate usage and availability to impact cerebral blood flow through both vasoconstriction and vasodilation. Interestingly, these opposite effects on the vascular tone involve different but parallel signaling cascades in astrocytes.

Briefly, neuronal release of glutamate can stimulate the metabotropic glutamate receptors (mGluR) on astrocytes. This in turn activates phospholipase C and increases intracellular calcium. Ca^{2+} transients in astrocytes activate cytosolic phospholipase A2 (PLA2), thus producing arachidonic acid (AA). AA can be used for the synthesis of prostaglandins, which can have different types of vasodilating effects. In parallel, AA can diffuse to arteriolar smooth muscle cells, where it is converted to 20-hydroxyeicosatetraenoic acid (20-HETE), which has a vasoconstricting effect. Whether the predominant impact on vascular tone is dilation or constriction depends on levels of lactate and adenosine in the extracellular space.

During brain activation, consistent with low O_2, an increase in lactate in the extracellular space will enhance vasodilation by assisting in the accumulation of prostaglandin E2 (PGE2). Elevated adenosine also enhances vasodilation but through an inhibitory effect on the synthesis of 20-HETE. This is an interesting observation and suggests that cerebral blood flow is largely controlled by glycolytic (vs. oxidative) metabolism and that increased cerebral blood flow correlates with elevations in lactate concentration (rather than O_2 consumption).

References and resources

Text

Bélanger, M., I. Allaman, and P. J. Magistretti. "Brain Energy Metabolism: Focus on Astrocyte–Neuron Metabolic Cooperation." *Cell Metabolism* 14, no. 6 (December 2011): 724–738, https://doi.org/10.1016/j.cmet.2011.08.016.

Le, T., and V. Bhushan. *First Aid for the USMLE Step* 1, 29th ed. New York: McGraw Hill Education, 2018, 87, 314–315.

Lieberman, M., and A. Peet, eds. *Marks' Basic Medical Biochemistry: A Clinical Approach*, 5th ed. Philadelphia: Wolters Kluwer Health/Lippincott Williams & Wilkins, 2018, Chapter 46: Metabolism of the Nervous System.

Magistretti, P. J., and I. Allaman. "A Cellular Perspective on Brain Energy Metabolism and Functional Imaging." *Neuron* 86, no. 4 (May 2015): 883–901, https://doi.org/10.1016/j.neuron.2015.03.035.

Figures

Figure 1.1: Potential fates of glucose oxidation. Magistretti, P. J., and I. Allaman. "A Cellular Perspective on Brain Energy Metabolism and Functional Imaging." *Neuron* 86, no. 4 (May 2015): 883–901, https://doi.org/10.1016/j.neuron.2015.03.035. Adapted under fair use.

Figure 1.2: Comparison of neuron andd astrocyte metabollism. Magistretti, P. J., and I. Allaman. "A Cellular Perspective on Brain Energy Metabolism and Functional Imaging." *Neuron* 86, no. 4 (May 2015): 883–901, https://doi.org/10.1016/j.neuron.2015.03.035. Adapted under fair use.

Figure 1.3: Lactate and glutamate shuttling between the astrocyte and neuron. Magistretti, P. J., and I. Allaman. "A Cellular Perspective on Brain Energy Metabolism and Functional Imaging." *Neuron* 86, no. 4 (May 2015): 883–901, https://doi.org/10.1016/j.neuron.2015.03.035. Adapted under fair use. Added diagram of an astrocyte by Cancer Research UK, CC BY 4.0., Wikimedia Commons, https://commons.wikimedia.org/wiki/F...1_CRUK_029.svg.

2. Neurotransmitters — ACh, glutamate, GABA, and glycine

Learning Objectives

- Define the characteristics of a classical neurotransmitter.
- Describe the synthetic pathways, inactivation mechanisms, and neurochemical anatomy and mechanisms of receptor transduction for the following classical and nonclassical neurotransmitters:
    - Acetylcholine
    - Glutamate
    - GABA (γ-aminobutyric acid)
    - Glycine
    - Catecholamines: dopamine, norepinephrine, epinephrine
    - Histamine
    - Serotonin (5-hydroxytryptaine)
- Review the major receptor classifications and representative receptor agonists and antagonists for the above transmitters.
- Compare steps of Gs protein activation versus steps that lead to an increase in intracellular Ca^{2+} and activation of protein kinase C following activation of a Gq protein.

Neurotransmitters are classically defined as:

1. Being located in the neuron and produced by the neuron;
2. Being released into the synaptic cleft when the neuron is stimulated;
3. Acting on a postsynaptic receptor when released and causing a biological effect; and
4. Being inactivated after they are released.

Acetylcholine

Acetylcholine (ACh) was the first identified neurotransmitter and is synthesized in nerve terminals from the precursors acetyl-CoA and choline, in a reaction catalyzed by choline acetyltransferase (ChAT) (figure 2.1). After synthesis in the cytoplasm of the neuron, a vesicular ACh transporter (VAChT) loads ACh into each cholinergic vesicle. The energy required to concentrate ACh within the vesicle is provided by the acidic pH of the vesicle lumen, which allows the VAChT to exchange H^+ for ACh.

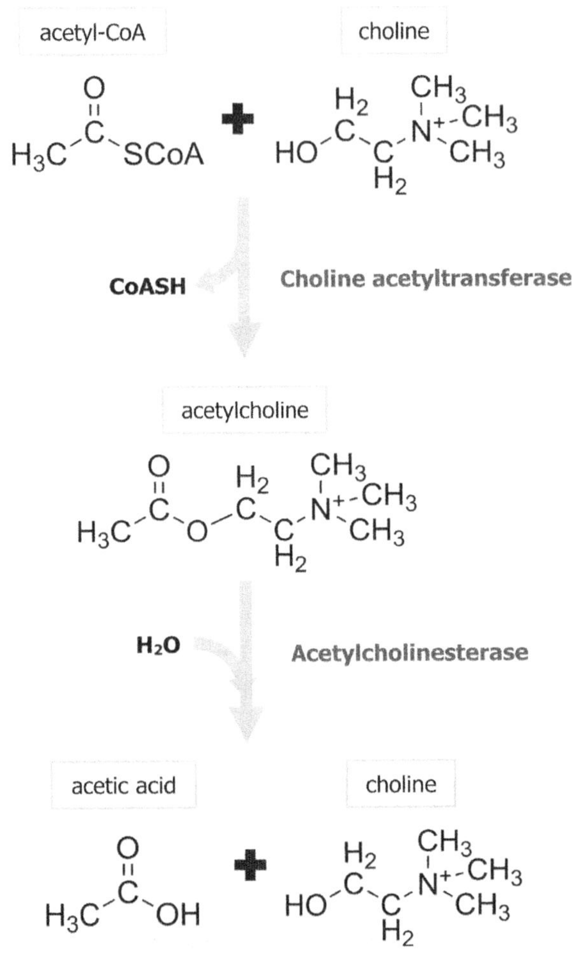

Figure 2.1: Synthesis and degradation of acetylcholine.

Termination of signal

In contrast to most other small-molecule neurotransmitters, the postsynaptic actions of ACh are not terminated by reuptake but hydrolysis by acetylcholinesterase (AChE). This enzyme is concentrated in the synaptic cleft, ensuring a rapid decrease in ACh concentration after its release from the presynaptic terminal. The hydrolysis results in acetate and choline (figure 2.1), which is recycled by being transported back into nerve terminals, where it is used to resynthesize ACh. Organophosphates are one class of drugs known to interact with ACh signal transmission through the inhibition of AChE, allowing ACh to accumulate at cholinergic synapses. This buildup of ACh depolarizes the postsynaptic muscle cell and renders it refractory to subsequent ACh release, causing neuromuscular paralysis.

Acetylcholine receptors

Many of the postsynaptic actions of ACh are mediated by the nicotinic ACh receptor (nAChR). nAChRs are nonselective cation channels that generate excitatory postsynaptic responses. Nicotinic receptors are large protein complexes consisting of five subunits. At the neuromuscular junction, the nAChR contains two α subunits, each of which has a binding site that binds a single molecule of ACh. Both ACh binding sites must be occupied for the receptor to be activated. In summary, the nAChR is a ligand-gated ion channel.

A second class of ACh receptors are referred to as muscarinic ACh receptors (mAChRs). mAChRs are metabotropic and mediate most of the effects of ACh in the brain. Like other metabotropic receptors, mAChRs have seven helical membrane-spanning domains. Binding of ACh to the receptor causes a conformational change that permits G-proteins to bind to the cytoplasmic domain of the mAChR (figure 2.2).

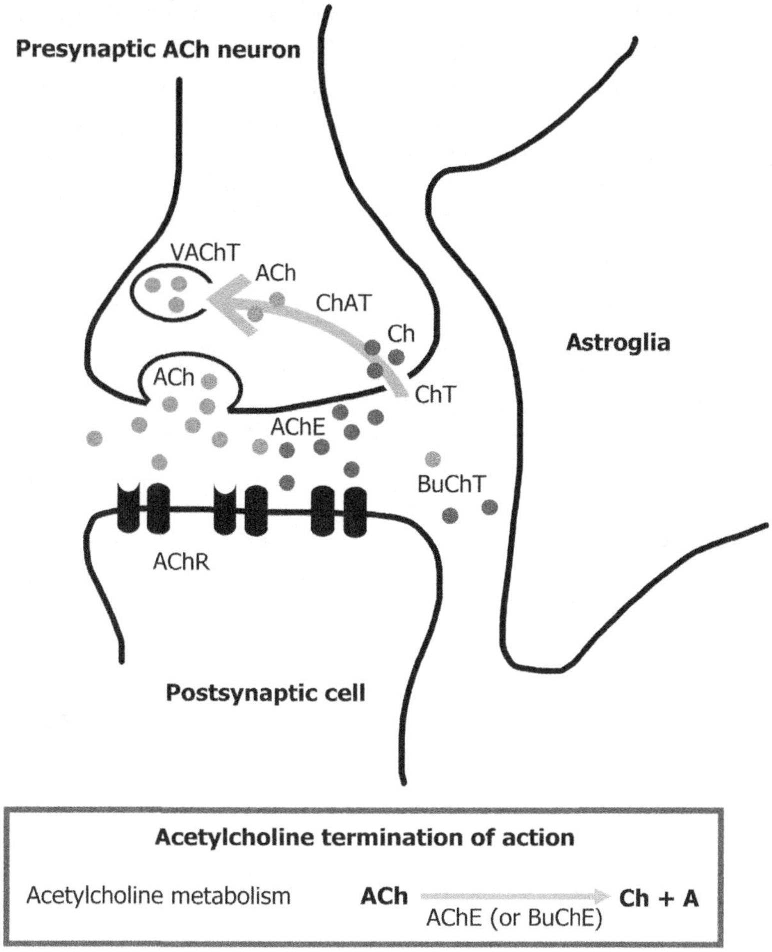

Figure 2.2: ACh release and degradation. (A: acetyl-CoA; ACh: acetylcholine; AChE: acetylcholine esterase; Ch: choline; VAChT: vesicular ACh transporter)

Glutamate

Glutamate is the most important transmitter for normal brain function. Nearly all excitatory neurons in the central nervous system (CNS) are glutamatergic. Glutamate is a nonessential amino acid that does not cross the blood-brain barrier and therefore must be synthesized in neurons from local precursors. The most prevalent precursor for glutamate synthesis is glutamine, which is taken up into presynaptic terminals by the system A transporter 2 (SAT2) and is then metabolized to glutamate by the mitochondrial enzyme glutaminase (figure 2.3).

Termination of signal

Glutamate synthesized in the presynaptic cytoplasm is packaged into synaptic vesicles by vesicular glutamate transporters (VGLUTs). Once released, glutamate is removed from the synaptic cleft by the excitatory amino acid transporters (EAATs). EAATs are a family of five different Na^+-dependent glutamate cotransporters. Some EAATs are present in glial cells and others in presynaptic terminals. Glutamate transported into glial cells via EAATs is converted into glutamine by the enzyme glutamine synthetase. Glutamine is then transported out of the glial cells by a different transporter, the system N transporter 1 (SN1), and transported into nerve terminals via SAT2. This overall sequence of events is referred to as the glutamate-glutamine cycle. This cycle allows glial cells and presynaptic terminals to cooperate both to maintain an adequate supply of glutamate for synaptic transmission and to rapidly terminate postsynaptic glutamate action (figure 2.4).

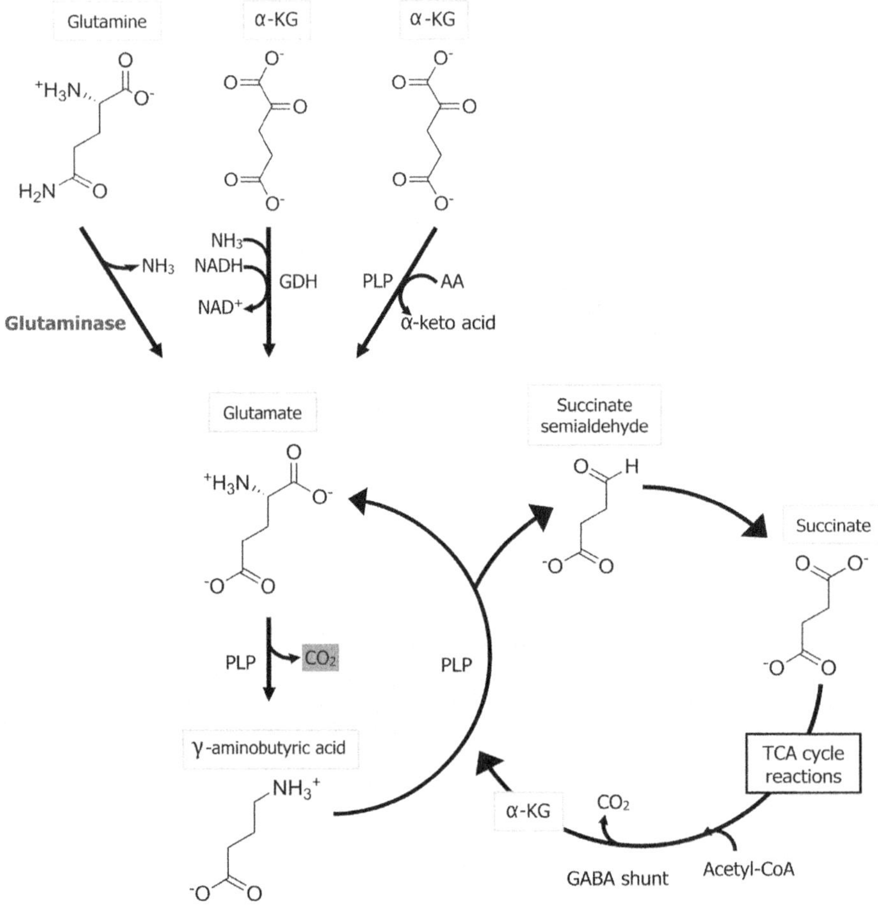

Figure 2.3: Glutamate and GABA synthesis. (α-KG: α-ketoglutarate; PLP: pyridoxal phosphate)

Glutamate receptors

There are several types of ionotropic glutamate receptors: AMPA receptors, NMDA receptors, and kainate receptors, named after the agonists that activate them: AMPA (α-amino-3-hydroxyl-5-methyl-4-isoxazole-propionate), NMDA (N-methyl-d-aspartate), and kainic acid. All of these receptors are glutamate-gated cation channels that allow the passage of Na^+ and K^+. Therefore AMPA, kainate, and NMDA receptor activation always produces excitatory postsynaptic responses. Most central excitatory synapses possess both AMPA and NMDA receptors. Antagonist drugs that selectively block either AMPA or NMDA receptors are often used to identify synaptic responses mediated by each receptor type. The physiological roles of kainate receptors are less well defined; in some cases, these receptors are found on presynaptic terminals and serve as a feedback mechanism to regulate glutamate release.

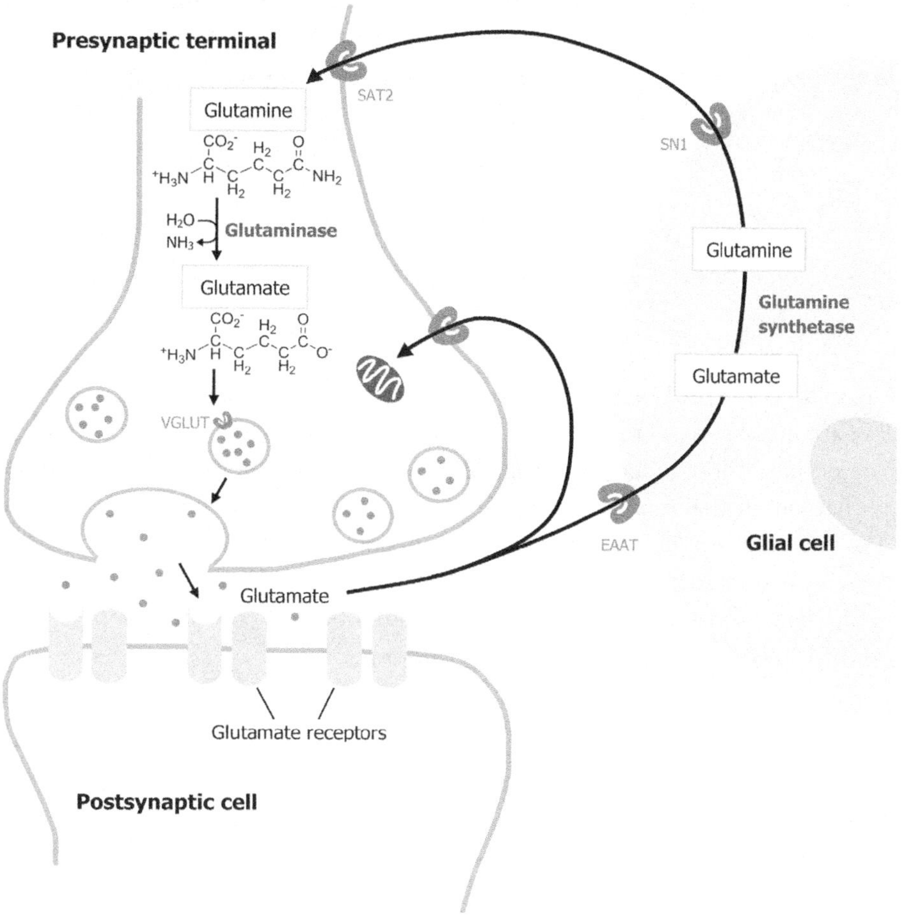

Figure 2.4: Glutamate release and reuptake. (EAAT: excitatory amino acid transporters)

In addition to these ionotropic glutamate receptors, there are three classes of metabotropic glutamate receptors (mGluRs). These receptors differ in their coupling to intracellular signal transduction pathways and in their sensitivity to pharmacological agents. Activation of many of these receptors leads to inhibition of postsynaptic Ca^{2+} and Na^{+} channels. Unlike the excitatory ionotropic glutamate receptors, mGluRs cause slower postsynaptic responses that can either excite or inhibit postsynaptic cells. As a result, the physiological roles of mGluRs are quite varied.

GABA

Most inhibitory synapses in the brain and spinal cord use either γ-aminobutyric acid (GABA) or glycine as neurotransmitters. The predominant precursor for GABA synthesis is glucose, which is metabolized to glutamate by the tricarboxylic acid cycle enzymes (figure 2.3). The enzyme glutamic acid decarboxylase (GAD), which is found almost exclusively in GABAergic neurons, catalyzes the conversion of glutamate to GABA. GAD requires pyridoxal phosphate for activity; a deficiency of this vitamin can lead to diminished GABA synthesis.

Termination of signal

Once GABA is synthesized, it is transported into synaptic vesicles via a vesicular inhibitory amino acid transporter (VIAAT). The mechanism of GABA removal is similar to that of glutamate. Both neurons and glia contain high-affinity Na^+-dependent cotransporters for GABA, and these cotransporters are termed GATs. Most GABA is eventually converted to succinate, which is metabolized further in the tricarboxylic acid cycle that mediates cellular ATP synthesis.

Two mitochondrial enzymes are required for this degradation: GABA transaminase and succinic semialdehyde dehydrogenase.

GABA receptors

GABAergic synapses employ two types of postsynaptic receptors, called $GABA_A$ and $GABA_B$. $GABA_A$ are ionotropic receptors, while $GABA_B$ are metabotropic receptors. The ionotropic $GABA_A$ receptors are GABA-gated anion channels, with Cl^- being the main permeant ion under physiological conditions. Thus, activation of these GABA receptors causes an influx of negatively charged Cl^- that inhibits postsynaptic cells. The same site binds the hypnotic zolpidem (Ambien), which is widely used to induce sleep. Barbiturates such as phenobarbital and pentobarbital are other hypnotics that also bind to the extracellular domains of the α and β subunits of some GABA receptors and potentiate GABAergic transmission; these drugs are used therapeutically for anesthesia and to control epilepsy. The injection anesthetic ketamine also binds to the extracellular domain of GABA receptors.

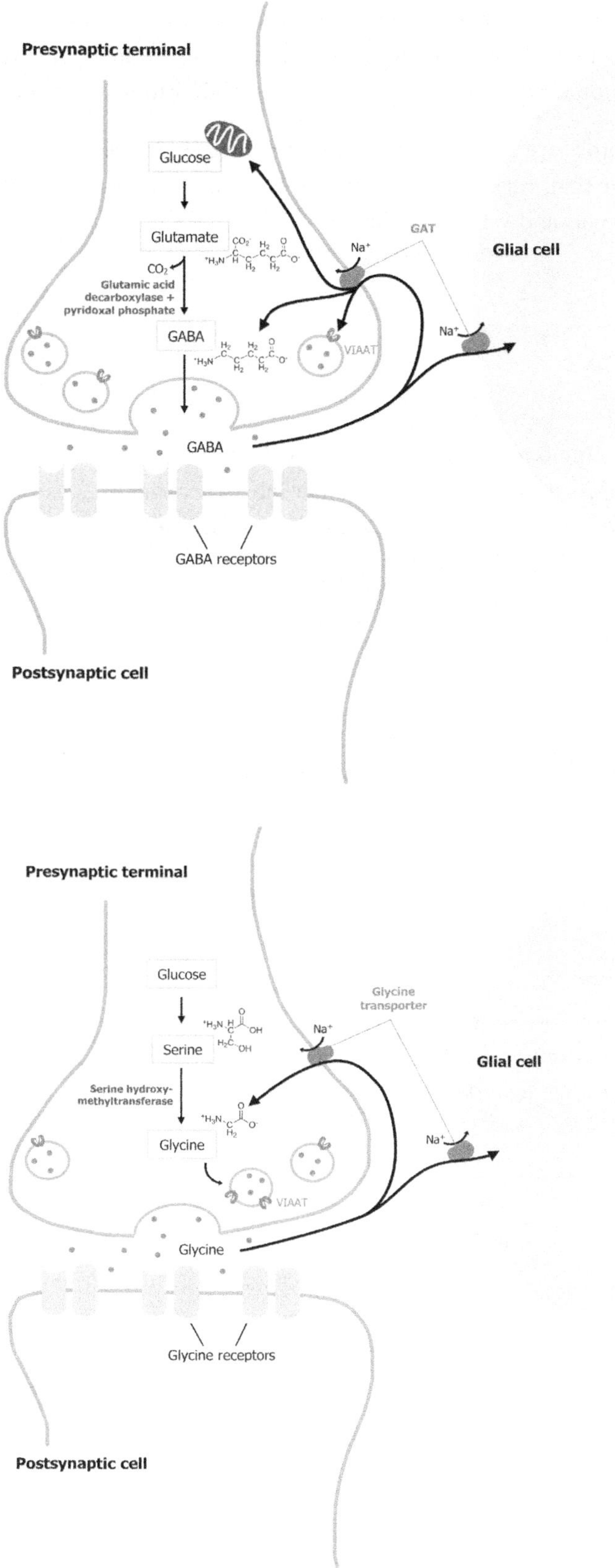

Figure 2.5: GABA and glycine release. (GAT: cotransporters for GABA; VIAAT: vesicular inhibitory amino acid transporter)

The transmembrane domains of $GABA_A$ receptors also serve as the targets for numerous ligands, such as inhalant anesthetics and steroids. Another drug that binds to the transmembrane domain of $GABA_A$ receptors is ethanol; at least some aspects of drunken behavior are caused by ethanol-mediated alterations in ionotropic GABA receptors.

The metabotropic $GABA_B$ receptors are also widely distributed in the brain. Like the ionotropic GABA receptors, $GABA_B$ receptors are inhibitory. Rather than relying on Cl^--selective channels, however, $GABA_B$-mediated inhibition is often due to the activation of K^+ channels and subsequent efflux of K^+.

Glycine

The distribution of the neutral amino acid glycine in the CNS is more restricted than that of GABA. About half of the inhibitory synapses in the spinal cord use glycine; most other inhibitory synapses use GABA. Glycine is synthesized from serine by the mitochondrial isoform of serine hydroxymethyltransferase (figure 2.5) and is transported into synaptic vesicles via the same VIAAT that loads GABA into vesicles.

Termination of signal

Once released from the presynaptic cell, glycine is rapidly removed from the synaptic cleft by glycine transporters in the plasma membrane (figure 2.5).

Glycine receptors

Glycine receptors are pentamers consisting of a combination of four types of α subunits, along with an accessory β subunit. These receptors are potently blocked by strychnine, which may account for the toxic properties of this plant alkaloid. Glycine receptors are ligand-gated Cl^- channels whose general structure closely mirrors that of the $GABA_A$ receptors.

Neurotransmitter	**Postsynaptic effect**	**Precursor(s)**	**Rate-limiting step**	**Removal mechanism**
ACh	Excitatory	Chlorine + acetyl-CoA	ChAT	ACh-esterase
Glutamate	Excitatory	Glutamine	Glutaminase	Transporters
GABA	Inhibitory	Glutamine	GAD	Transporters
Glycine	Inhibitory	Serine	Phosphoserine	Transporters

2.1: Acetylcholine and the primary amino acid neurotransmitters.

Biogenic amines

Biogenic amine transmitters regulate many brain functions and are also active in the peripheral nervous system. There are five well-established biogenic amine neurotransmitters, three of which can be classified as catecholamines:

1. Dopamine (catecholamine),
2. Adrenaline/noradrenaline (catecholamine),
3. Epinephrine/norepinephrine (catecholamine),
4. Histamine, and
5. Serotonin.

Dopamine

The first step in catecholamine synthesis is catalyzed by tyrosine hydroxylase in a reaction requiring oxygen as a cosubstrate and tetrahydrobiopterin as a cofactor to synthesize dihydroxyphenylalanine (DOPA) (figure 2.6).

Dopamine is produced by the action of DOPA decarboxylase on DOPA. Following its synthesis in the cytoplasm of presynaptic terminals, dopamine is loaded into synaptic vesicles via a vesicular monoamine transporter (VMAT). Dopamine action in the synaptic cleft is terminated by reuptake of dopamine into nerve terminals or surrounding glial cells by a Na^+-dependent dopamine cotransporter, termed DAT.

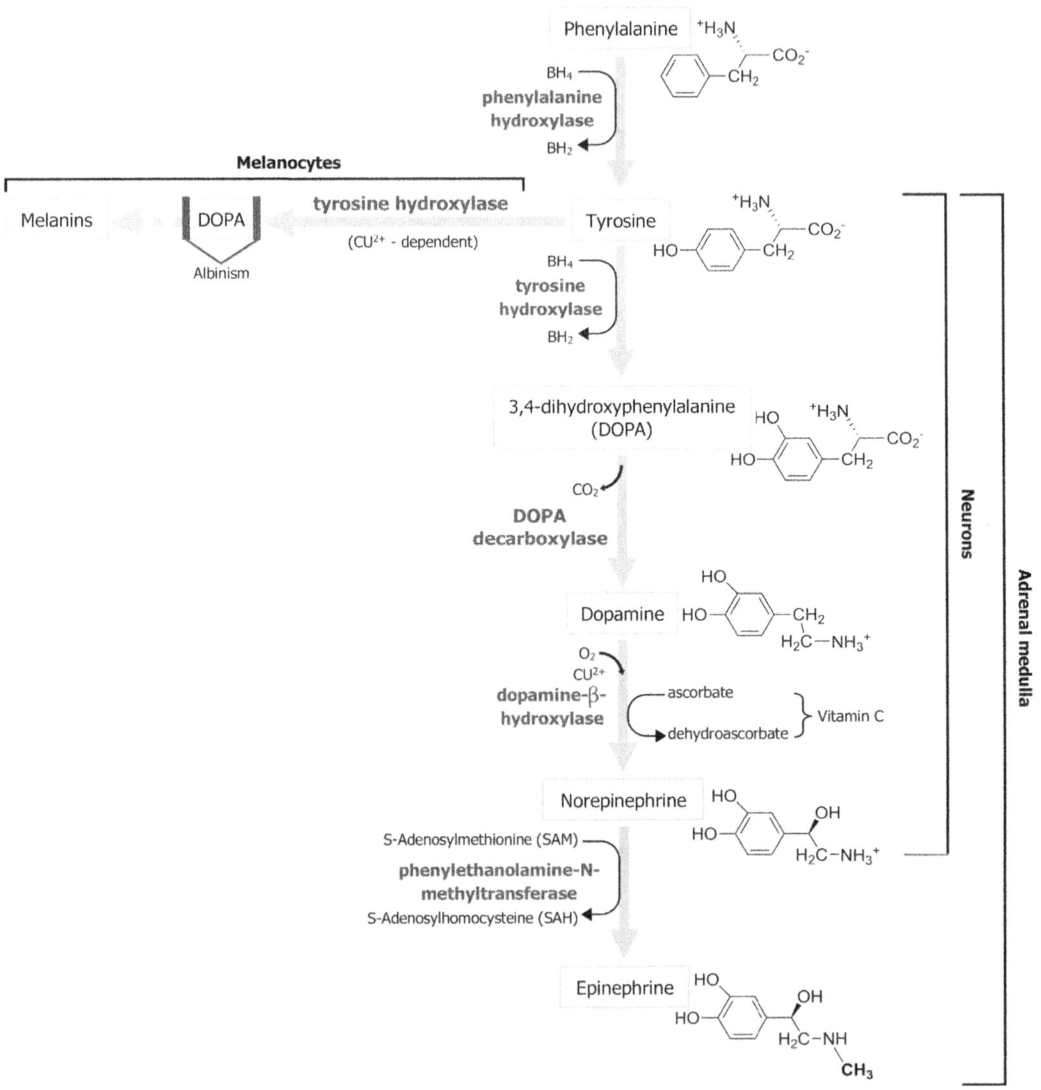

Figure 2.6: Synthesis of dopamine, norepinephrine, and epinephrine.

Termination of signal

The two major enzymes involved in the catabolism of dopamine are monoamine oxidase (MAO) and catechol O-methyltransferase (COMT). Both neurons and glia contain mitochondrial MAO and cytoplasmic COMT.

Dopamine receptors

Once released, dopamine acts exclusively by activating G-protein–coupled receptors. Most dopamine receptor subtypes act by either activating or inhibiting adenylyl cyclase. Activation of these receptors generally contributes to complex behaviors.

Norepinephrine (also called noradrenaline) is used as a neurotransmitter and influences sleep and wakefulness, arousal, attention, and feeding behavior. Perhaps the most prominent noradrenergic neurons are sympathetic ganglion cells, which employ norepinephrine as the major peripheral transmitter in this division of the visceral motor system.

Norepinephrine synthesis requires dopamine β-hydroxylase, which catalyzes the production of norepinephrine from dopamine (figure 2.6). Norepinephrine is then loaded into synaptic vesicles via the same VMAT involved in vesicular dopamine transport.

Termination of signal

Norepinephrine is cleared from the synaptic cleft by the norepinephrine transporter (NET), an Na^+-dependent cotransporter that is also capable of taking up dopamine. NET is a molecular target of amphetamine, which acts as a stimulant by producing a net increase in the release of norepinephrine and dopamine. Like dopamine, norepinephrine is degraded by MAO and COMT.

Epinephrine (also called adrenaline) is found in the brain at lower levels than the other catecholamines and is also present in fewer brain neurons than other catecholamines. Epinephrine-secreting neurons regulate respiration and cardiac function. The enzyme that synthesizes epinephrine, phenylethanolamine-N-methyltransferase (figure 2.6), is present only in epinephrine-secreting neurons. Otherwise, the metabolism of epinephrine is very similar to that of norepinephrine. Epinephrine is loaded into vesicles via the VMAT. No plasma membrane transporter specific for epinephrine has been identified, although the NET is capable of transporting epinephrine. As already noted, epinephrine acts on both α- and β-adrenergic receptors.

Epinephrine and norepinephrine signaling

Both norepinephrine and epinephrine act on α- and β-adrenergic receptors. Both types of receptor are G-protein-coupled; in fact, the β-adrenergic receptor was the first identified metabotropic neurotransmitter receptor. Binding of norepinephrine or epinephrine causes small changes in the structure of this receptor, which permits the G-protein to bind. This, in turn, causes larger changes in the shape of the α subunit of the G-protein, the first step in a series of reactions that allow the G-protein to regulate intracellular signaling cascades.

Two subclasses of α-adrenergic receptors have been identified. Activation of α1 – *adernergic* receptors usually results in a slow depolarization linked to the inhibition of K^+ channels, while activation of α2 receptors produces a slow hyperpolarization due to the activation of a different type of K^+ channel. There are three subtypes of β-adrenergic receptors, two of which are expressed in many types of neurons.

Histamine

Histamine is found in neurons in the hypothalamus that send sparse but widespread projections to almost all regions of the brain and spinal cord. The central histamine projections mediate arousal and attention, similar to central ACh and norepinephrine projections. Histamine also controls the reactivity of the vestibular system. Allergic reactions or tissue damage cause release of histamine from mast cells in the bloodstream. The close proximity of mast cells to blood vessels, together with the potent actions of histamine on blood vessels, raises the possibility that histamine may influence brain blood flow.

Histamine is produced from the amino acid histidine by a histidine decarboxylase (figure 2.7) and is transported into vesicles via the same VMAT as the catecholamines. No plasma membrane histamine transporter has been identified yet.

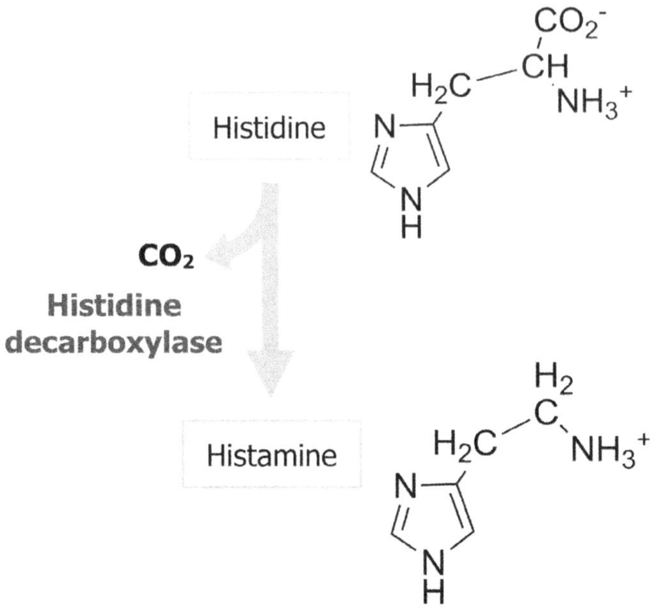

Figure 2.7: Histamine synthesis.

Termination of signal

Histamine is degraded by the combined actions of histamine methyltransferase and MAO.

Histamine receptors

The four known types of histamine receptors are all metabotropic receptors. Of the four, only two of the receptors (H_1 and H_2) are well characterized. Because of the role of histamine receptors in mediating allergic responses, many histamine receptor antagonists have been developed as antihistamine agents. Antihistamines that cross the blood-brain barrier, such as diphenhydramine (Benadryl), act as sedatives by interfering with the roles of histamine in CNS arousal. Antagonists of the H_1 receptor also are used to prevent motion sickness, perhaps because of the role of histamine in controlling vestibular function (figure 2.8).

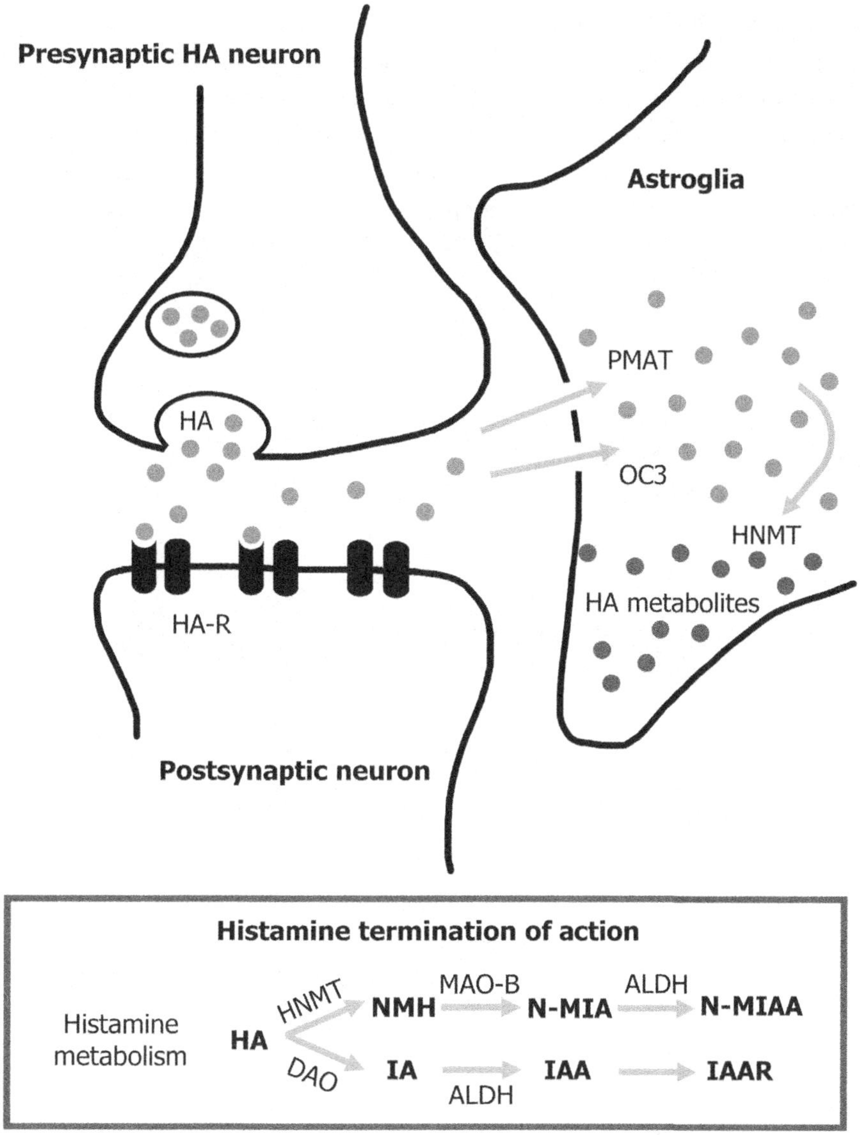

Figure 2.8: Histamine release and reuptake. (ALDH: *aldehyde dehydrogenase*; DAO: *diamine oxidase*; HA: *histamine*; HNMT: N-*methyltransferase*; IA: *imidazole acetaldehyde*; IAA: *imidazoleacetic acid*; IAAR: *imidazoleacetic acid riboside*; NMH: N-*methylhistamine*; N-MIA: *methylimidazole acetaldehyde*; N-MIAA: N-*methylimidazoleacetic acetic acid*; OC3: *organic cation transporter 3*; PMAT: *plasma membrane monoamine transporter*)

H_2 receptors control the secretion of gastric acid in the digestive system, allowing H_2 receptor antagonists to be used in treating a variety of upper gastrointestinal disorders (e.g., peptic ulcers).

Serotonin

Serotonin, or 5-hydroxytryptamine (5-HT), was initially thought to increase vascular tone by virtue of its presence in blood serum (hence the name serotonin). 5-HT is synthesized from the amino acid tryptophan, which is an essential dietary requirement. Tryptophan is taken up into neurons by a plasma membrane transporter and hydroxylated in a reaction catalyzed by the enzyme tryptophan-5-hydroxylase (figure 2.9), the rate-limiting step for 5-HT synthesis. Loading of 5-HT into synaptic vesicles is done by the VMAT that is also responsible for loading other monoamines into synaptic vesicles. The synaptic effects of serotonin are terminated by transport back into nerve terminals via a specific serotonin transporter (SERT) that is present in the presynaptic plasma membrane and is encoded by the 5HTT gene. Many antidepressant drugs are selective serotonin reuptake inhibitors (SSRIs) that inhibit transport of 5-HT by SERT. Perhaps the best-known example of an SSRI is the antidepressant drug Prozac.

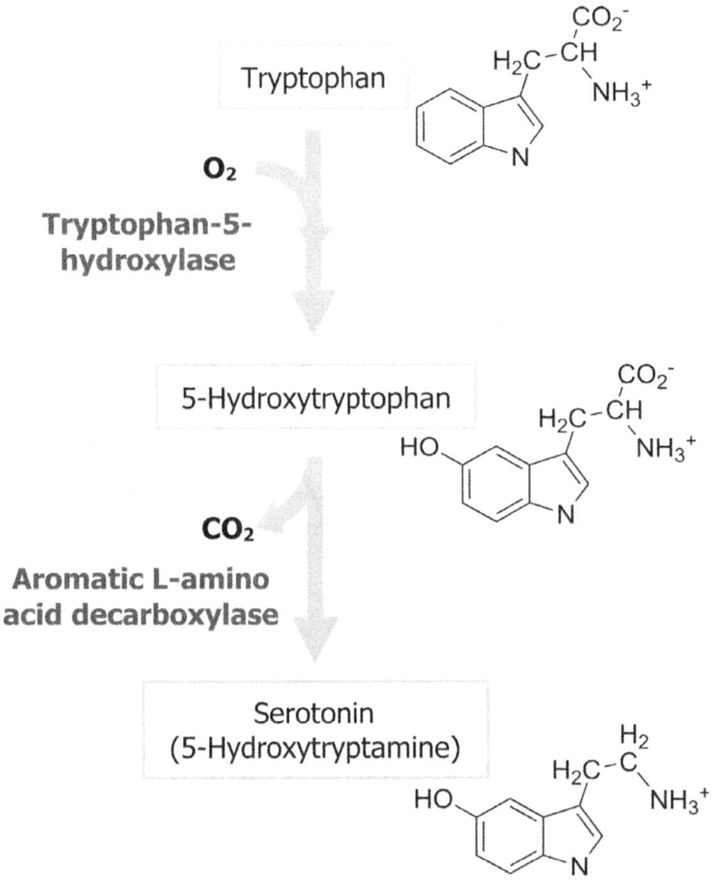

Figure 2.9: Serotonin synthesis.

Termination of signal

The primary catabolic pathway for 5-HT is mediated by MAO.

Serotonin receptors

Most 5-HT receptors are metabotropic, with a monomeric structure typical of G-protein–coupled receptors. Metabotropic 5-HT receptors have been implicated in a wide range of behaviors, including circadian rhythms, motor behaviors, emotional states, and mental arousal. Impairments in the function of these receptors have been implicated in numerous psychiatric disorders, such as depression, anxiety disorders, and schizophrenia, and drugs acting on serotonin receptors are effective treatments for several of these conditions.

Neurotransmitter	Postsynaptic effect	Precursor(s)	Rate-limiting step	Removal mechanism
ACh	Excitatory	Choline + acetyl-CoA	ChAT	ACh-esterase
Glutamate	Excitatory	Glutamine	Glutaminase	Transporters
GABA	Inhibitory	Glutamine	GAD	Transporters
Glycine	Inhibitory	Serine	Phosphoserine	Transporters
Catecholamines (dopamine, epi, norepi)	Excitatory	Tyrosine	Tyrosine hydroxylase	MAO; COMT
Histamine	Excitatory	Histidine	Histidine decarboxylase	Transporters
Serotonin (5-HT)	Excitatory	Tryptophan	Tryptophan hydroxylase	MAO; COMT

Table 2.2: Summary of neurotransmitter synthesis and degradation.

References and resources

Text

"Biochemistry of Nerve Transmission." The Medical Biochemistry Page. http://themedicalbiochemistrypage.or...-transmission/.

"Neurotransmitters and Receptors: Different Classes of Neurotransmitters, and Different Types of Receptors They Bind To." Khan Academy. https://www.khanacademy.org/science/...heir-receptors.

Purves, D., G. J. Augustine, Dd. Fitzpatrick, L. C. Katz, A.-S. LaMantia, J. O. McNamara, and S. M. Williams, eds. *Neuroscience*, 2nd ed. Sunderland, MA: Sinauer Associates, 2001, Chapter 6: Neurotransmitters.

Figures

Figure 2.1: Synthesis and degradation of acetylcholine. Grey, Kindred. "Synthesis and Degradation of Acetylcholine." 2021, https://archive.org/details/2.1_20210817. CC BY 4.0. Chemical structure by Henry Jakubowski.

Figure 2.2: ACh release and degradation. Grey, Kindred. "ACh Release and Degradation." 2021, https://archive.org/details/2.2_20210817. CC BY 4.0. Added curved left arrow by Star and Anchor Design from the Noun Project.

Figure 2.3: Glutamate and GABA synthesis. Lieberman, M., and A. Peet, eds. *Marks' Basic Medical Biochemistry: A Clinical Approach*, 5th ed. Philadelphia: Wolters Kluwer Health/Lippincott Williams & Wilkins, 2018, 747, Figure 35.7: The gama glutamyl cycle. Adapted under fair use. Chemical structure by Henry Jakubowski.

Figure 2.4: Glutamate release and reuptake. Purves, D., G. J. Augustine, D. Fitzpatrick, W. C. Hall, A.-S. LaMantia, R. D. Mooney, M. L. Platt, and L. E. White. *Neuroscience*, 6th ed. New York: Oxford University Press, 2017, 122, Figure 6.5: Glutamate synthesis and cycling between neurons and glia. Adapted under fair use. Added beans by Vectors Market from the Noun Project. Chemical structure by Henry Jakubowski.

Figure 2.5: GABA and glycine release. Purves, D., G. J. Augustine, D. Fitzpatrick, W. C. Hall, A.-S. LaMantia, R. D. Mooney, M. L. Platt, and L. E. White. *Neuroscience*, 6th ed. New York: Oxford University Press, 2017, 127, Figure 6.10: Synthesis, release and reuptake of the inhibitor neurotransmitters GABA and glycine. Adapted under fair use. Added beans by Vectors Market from the Noun Project. Chemical structure by Henry Jakubowski.

Figure 2.6: Synthesis of dopamine, norepinephrine, and epinephrine. Grey, Kindred. "Synthesis of Dopamine, Norepinephrine and Epinephrine. 2021, https://archive.org/details/2.6_20210819. CC BY 4.0. Chemical structure by Henry Jakubowski.

Figure 2.7: Histamine synthesis. Purves, D., G. J. Augustine, D. Fitzpatrick, W. C. Hall, A.-S. LaMantia, R. D. Mooney, M. L. Platt, and L. E. White. *Neuroscience*, 6th ed. New York: Oxford University Press, 2017, 134, Figure 6.18: Synthesis of histamine and serotonin. Adapted under fair use. Chemical structure by Henry Jakubowski.

Figure 2.8: Histamine release and reuptake. Grey, Kindred. "Histamine Release and Reuptake." 2021, https://archive.org/details/2.8_20210819. CC BY 4.0.

Figure 2.9: Serotonin synthesis. Purves, D., G. J. Augustine, D. Fitzpatrick, W. C. Hall, A.-S. LaMantia, R. D. Mooney, M. L. Platt, and L. E. White. *Neuroscience*, 6th ed. New York: Oxford University Press, 2017, 134, Figure 6.18: Synthesis of histamine and serotonin. Adapted under fair use. Chemical structure by Henry Jakubowski.

3. Neuropeptides and unconventional neurotransmitters

Learning Objectives

- Describe the synthetic pathways, inactivation mechanisms, and neurochemical anatomy and mechanisms of receptor transduction for the following nonclassical neurotransmitters:
    - Substance P
    - Opioid peptides
    - Endocannabinoids
    - Nitric oxide
    - Carbon monoxide
    - ATP
    - Adenosine
- Review the major receptor classifications and representative receptor agonists and antagonists for the above transmitters.

Many biological peptide hormones also act as neurotransmitters. Neurotransmitters modulate a host of responses with some peptide transmitters implicated in modulating emotions, while others, such as substance P, are involved in the perception of pain. Additional peptides, such as melanocyte-stimulating hormones, adrenocorticotropin, and β-endorphin, regulate complex responses to stress, feeding behaviors, and anxiety.

The mechanisms responsible for the synthesis and packaging of peptide transmitters are distinct from those used for the small-molecule neurotransmitters but have similarities to the processes used for the synthesis of proteins that are secreted from nonneuronal cells (pancreatic enzymes).

Peptide neurotransmitters

Peptide-secreting neurons generally synthesize polypeptides that are much larger than the final, "mature" peptide. Processing these polypeptides, which are called pre-propeptides, takes place within the neuron's cell body by a sequence of reactions that occur in several intracellular organelles. Pre-propeptides are synthesized in the rough endoplasmic reticulum, where the signal sequence—that is, the sequence of amino acids indicating that the peptide is to be secreted—is removed. The remaining polypeptide, referred to as the propeptide, moves through the Golgi apparatus and is packaged into vesicles in the trans-Golgi network. The final stages of peptide neurotransmitter processing involve proteolytic cleavage and occur within the Golgi-associated vesicles. In addition to cleavage, modification of the ends of the peptide by glycosylation, phosphorylation, and disulfide bond formation is also common.

Neuropeptides often are coreleased with small-molecule neurotransmitters. Thus, peptidergic synapses often elicit complex postsynaptic responses. Following release, these neuropeptides are inactivated into amino acid fragments by enzymes called peptidases that are typically located on the extracellular surface of the plasma membrane.

The biological activity of the peptide neurotransmitters depends on their amino acid sequence. Based on their sequences, neuropeptide transmitters have been loosely grouped into five categories:

1. Brain/gut peptides,
2. Opioid peptides,
3. Pituitary peptides,
4. Hypothalamic releasing hormones, and
5. Catch-all category containing "other."

Substance P is an eleven-amino-acid peptide classified as a brain/gut peptide due to its expression in both the human hippocampus and neocortex and gastrointestinal tract. It is also released from C fibers—afferents in peripheral nerves that convey information about pain and temperature.

Substance P is a sensory neurotransmitter in the spinal cord, where its release can be inhibited by opioid peptides released from spinal cord interneurons, resulting in the suppression of pain.

Opioid peptides were initially discovered in the 1970s while screening for endorphins, or endogenous compounds that mimicked the actions of morphine. The endogenous ligands of the opioid receptors have been identified and fall into three classes: endorphins, enkephalins, and dynorphins.

Each ligand is synthesized in an inactive pre-propeptide derived from distinct genes. Opioid precursor processing is tissue-specific and carried out within the Golgi apparatus.

Opioid peptides are often colocalized with neurotransmitters, such as GABA and 5-HT, and are found widely distributed in many regions of the brain. In general, opioids tend to be depressants. Opioids are also involved in more complex behaviors such as sexual attraction and aggressive and submissive behaviors. They have also been implicated in psychiatric disorders such as schizophrenia and autism, although the evidence for this is debated. Repeated administration of opioids can lead to tolerance, addiction, or dependence; therefore therapeutic use is highly regulated. There are three well-characterized opioid receptor subtypes (μ, δ, and κ) that play a role in reward mechanisms as well as addiction.

Neuropeptide receptors

Virtually all neuropeptides initiate their effects by activating G-protein-coupled receptors, however, studying these metabotropic peptide receptors in the brain has been difficult as there are few known specific agonists and antagonists. Neuropeptide receptor activation is important for a variety of homeostatic responses such as regulating the postganglionic output from sympathetic ganglia and the activity of the gut. Other peptide receptors, such as the neuropeptide Y receptor, are also involved in the initiation and maintenance of feeding behaviors that can lead to satiety or obesity, depending on regulation. Additional behaviors attributed to activation of peptide receptors include anxiety and panic attacks. These responses can be addressed through the use of antagonists of cholecystokinin receptors.

Unconventional neurotransmitters

There are also some unusual molecules that are used for signaling between neurons and their targets. These chemical signals can be considered as neurotransmitters because of their roles in interneuronal signaling and because their release from neurons is regulated by Ca^{2+}. However, they are unconventional in comparison with other neurotransmitters because:

1. They are not stored in synaptic vesicles.
2. They are not released from presynaptic terminals via exocytotic mechanisms.
3. They may not be released from presynaptic terminals at all and are often associated with retrograde signaling (that is, from postsynaptic cells back to presynaptic terminals).

Endocannabinoids are a family of related endogenous signals that interact with cannabinoid receptors. These receptors are the molecular targets of Δ9-tetrahydrocannabinol, the psychoactive component of the marijuana plant.

Production of endocannabinoids is stimulated by:

1. A second messenger within postsynaptic neurons, typically a rise in postsynaptic Ca^{2+} concentration.
2. This allows these hydrophobic signals to diffuse through the postsynaptic membrane to reach cannabinoid receptors on other nearby cells.
3. Endocannabinoid action is terminated by carrier-mediated transport of these signals back into the postsynaptic neuron, where they are hydrolyzed by the enzyme fatty acid hydrolase (FAAH).

At least two types of cannabinoid receptors have been identified, with most actions of endocannabinoids in the CNS. The CB1 receptor is a G-protein–coupled receptor related to the metabotropic receptors for ACh, glutamate, and other conventional neurotransmitters.

Nitric oxide (NO) is an unusual and especially interesting chemical signal. It is a gas produced by the action of nitric oxide synthase, an enzyme that converts the amino acid arginine into a metabolite (citrulline) and simultaneously generates NO.

Within neurons, NO synthase is regulated by Ca^{2+} binding to the Ca^{2+} sensor protein calmodulin. Once produced, NO can permeate the plasma membrane and act inside nearby cells. Thus, this gaseous signal has a range of influence that extends well beyond the cell of origin. This property makes NO a potentially useful agent for coordinating the activities of multiple cells in a localized region and may mediate certain forms of synaptic plasticity that spread within small networks of neurons.

All of the known actions of NO are mediated within its cellular targets; for this reason, NO often is considered a second messenger rather than a neurotransmitter. Some of the actions of NO are due to the activation of the enzyme guanylyl cyclase, which then produces the second messenger cGMP within target cells. Due to the gaseous nature of NO, termination of signal is difficult to characterize; NO will diffuse and the reduction in concentration is a likely termination.

Carbon monoxide (CO) is generated in neurons by the enzymatic cleavage of heme by heme oxygenase-2. CO binds hemoglobin and binds enzymes within the electron transport chain, however, in the case of the neuron, it is part of the neurovascular coupling mechanism and increases local vasodilation.

ATP and other purines

All synaptic vesicles contain ATP, which is coreleased with one or more "classical" neurotransmitters. It has been known since the 1920s that the extracellular application of ATP (or its breakdown products AMP and adenosine) can elicit electrical responses in neurons.

ATP acts as an excitatory neurotransmitter in motor neurons of the spinal cord, as well as in sensory and autonomic ganglia. Extracellular enzymes degrade released ATP to adenosine, which has its own set of signaling actions. Thus, adenosine cannot be considered a classical neurotransmitter because it is not stored in synaptic vesicles or released in a Ca^{2+}-dependent manner. Several enzymes are involved in the rapid catabolism and removal of purines from extracellular locations. Receptors for both ATP and adenosine are widely distributed in the nervous system as well as in many other tissues. There are three classes of these purinergic receptors. One class consists of ionotropic receptors called P2X receptors. The structure of these receptors is unique among ionotropic receptors because each subunit has a transmembrane domain that crosses the membrane only twice. The other two classes of purinergic receptors, P2Y, are G-protein-coupled metabotropic receptors. The two classes differ in their sensitivity to agonists—one type is preferentially stimulated by adenosine, whereas the other is preferentially activated by ATP.

References and resources

Text

Purves, D., G. J. Augustine, Dd. Fitzpatrick, L. C. Katz, A.-S. LaMantia, J. O. McNamara, and S. M. Williams, eds. *Neuroscience*, 2nd ed. Sunderland, MA: Sinauer Associates, 2001, Chapter 6: Neurotransmitters.

4. Amino acid metabolism and specialized products

Learning Objectives

- Define essential, conditionally essential, and nonessential amino acids, and explain how certain nonessential amino acids become essential in certain conditions.
- Integrate amino acid synthesis with specific precursors from glycolysis, the citric acid cycle, and the pentose phosphate pathway.
- Identify key roles of amino acids as substrates for the synthesis of specialized products, including heme, GABA, carnitine, glutathione, serotonin, histamine, ubiquinone, melanin, creatine, and dopamine.
- Review the role of transamination in the interconversion of amino acids and connection to the urea cycle.
- Distinguish the following disease states associated with inborn errors of metabolism, including (A) the deficient enzyme, (B) inheritance pattern of the disease, and (C) relation of the deficiency to the buildup of secondary metabolites. The following is a list of diseases to focus on:
    - Phenylketonuria (Phenylalanine metabolism)
    - Homocystinuria (Methionine metabolism)
    - Maple syrup urine disease (Branched-chain amino acid metabolism)
    - Alkaptouria (Tyrosine metabolism)

There are twenty amino acids required for metabolic homeostasis. Of the twenty amino acids, eleven are considered nonessential, meaning they can be synthesized by the body. With the exceptions of tyrosine and cysteine, nonessential amino acids can be synthesized from glucose and a nitrogen donor. The other nine amino acids are essential and must be supplied by the diet. In addition to supplying carbon for gluconeogenesis, amino acids play important roles in the synthesis of essential cellular components. Disruptions of many of these pathways can lead to clinical disorders, many of which are identified during newborn screenings. The synthesis of all amino acids will not be addressed in this section; rather the most clinically relevant pathways will be focused on.

Cofactors essential for amino acid metabolism

The metabolism of many amino acids largely relies on the availability of the cofactors pyridoxal phosphate (B_6 or PLP), tetrahydrobiopterin (BH_4), and tetrahydrofolate (TH_4). It is important to recognize that deficiencies in these cofactors could present in a similar manner as enzymatic deficiencies of specific pathways.

Pyridoxal phosphate (B_6 or PLP)

All transamination reactions require PLP as a cofactor. These reactions are essential for moving (or donating) ammonia from an amino acid to a keto-acid to generate a different amino acid.

Tetrahydrobiopterin (BH_4)

BH_4 is a cofactor synthesized from GTP. It is oxidized during hydroxylation reactions, most notably the conversion of phenylalanine to tyrosine. Enzymatic deficiencies leading to decreased synthesis of BH_4 can present similar to deficiencies in phenylalanine metabolism.

Tetrahydrofolate (FH_4)

Folate can exist in many forms and is often referred to as tetrahydrofolate. FH_4 is often found in various forms with a one-carbon group attached. These one-carbon groups, which make up the one-carbon pool, can be oxidized or reduced. One-carbon groups can be transferred to other compounds and play essential roles in the synthesis of glycine from serine, the synthesis of the base thymine (required for DNA synthesis), the purine bases required for both DNA and RNA synthesis, and the transfer of methyl groups to vitamin B_{12}.

Synthesis of specialized products

The following highlights some of the key aspects of amino acid metabolism.

Phenylalanine and tyrosine

Phenylalanine (Phe) is an essential amino acid, and hydroxylation of Phe by phenylalanine hydroxylase (PAH) generates tyrosine (figure 4.1). This conversion requires BH_4, and deficiencies in either the cofactor or the enzyme PAH can result in phenylketonuria. Additionally, the inability to synthesize tyrosine will make this a conditionally essential amino acid and potentially negatively impact the synthesis of downstream compounds illustrated in figure 4.2.

Tyrosine can be produced from phenylalanine metabolism and is required for the production of melanin and the catecholamines. Deficiencies can occur at several different locations in the pathway and result in albinism (tyrosinase), alkaptonuria (homogentisate oxidase), or tyrosinemia, which can manifest due to deficiencies in several enzymes along the pathway (figure 4.1).

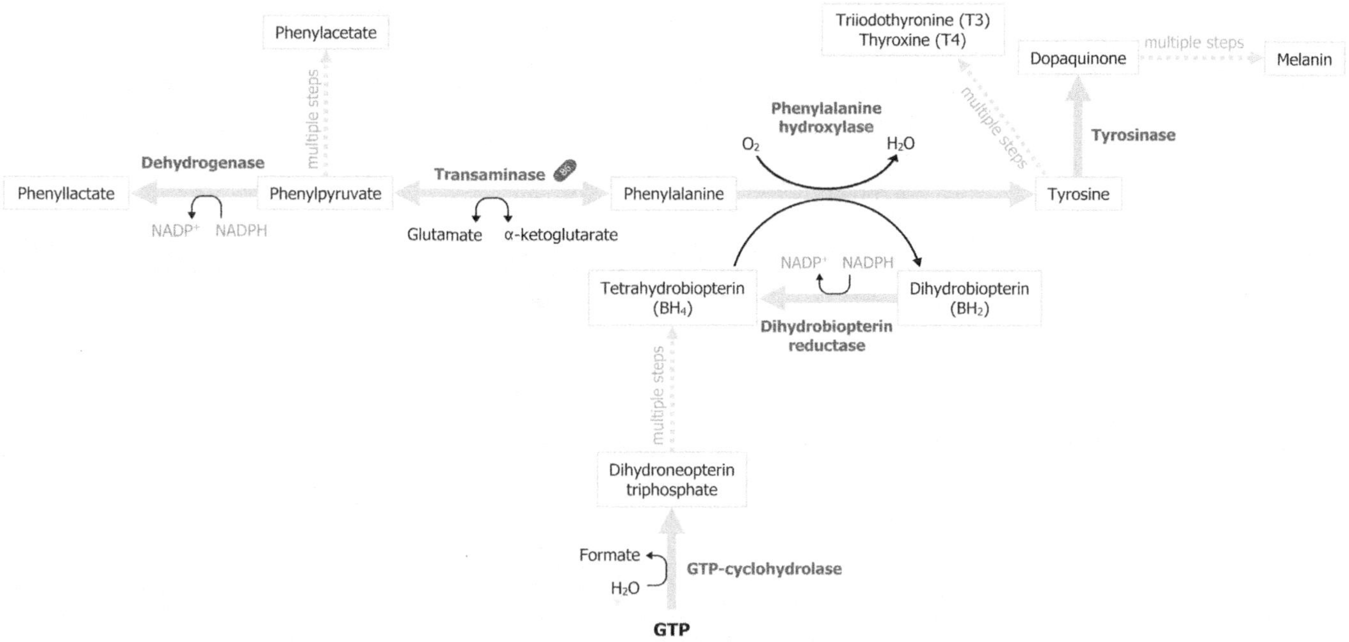

Figure 4.1: Metabolism of phenylalanine requires BH4 and also produces tyrosine. Deficiencies in cofactor or phenylalanine hydroxylase can result in phenylketonuria.

Phenylketonuria

Phenylketonuria (PKU) is one of the more common amino acid metabolic disorders and is inherited in an autosomal recessive fashion. There are no symptoms of untreated phenylketonuria in the first months of life. Therefore newborn screening is essential for diagnosis and initiation of treatment, which prevents the devastating effects of infantile hyperphenylalaninemia. The screening method detects elevated titers of the amino acid phenylalanine in the blood. A positive test result (Phe greater than 150 μmol/L) prompts the physician to begin a phenylalanine-restricted formula and requires a confirmatory quantitative Phe level.

Glycine

Glycine is a key compound that functions as an essential substrate for various pathways, including the folate cycle, nucleotide synthesis, and synthesis of porphyrins (heme), glutathione, and creatine.

Arginine

Arginine is a nonessential amino acid as it can be produced in the urea cycle. Deficiencies in the urea cycle can cause arginine to become conditionally essential. In these cases, management and supplementation are needed.

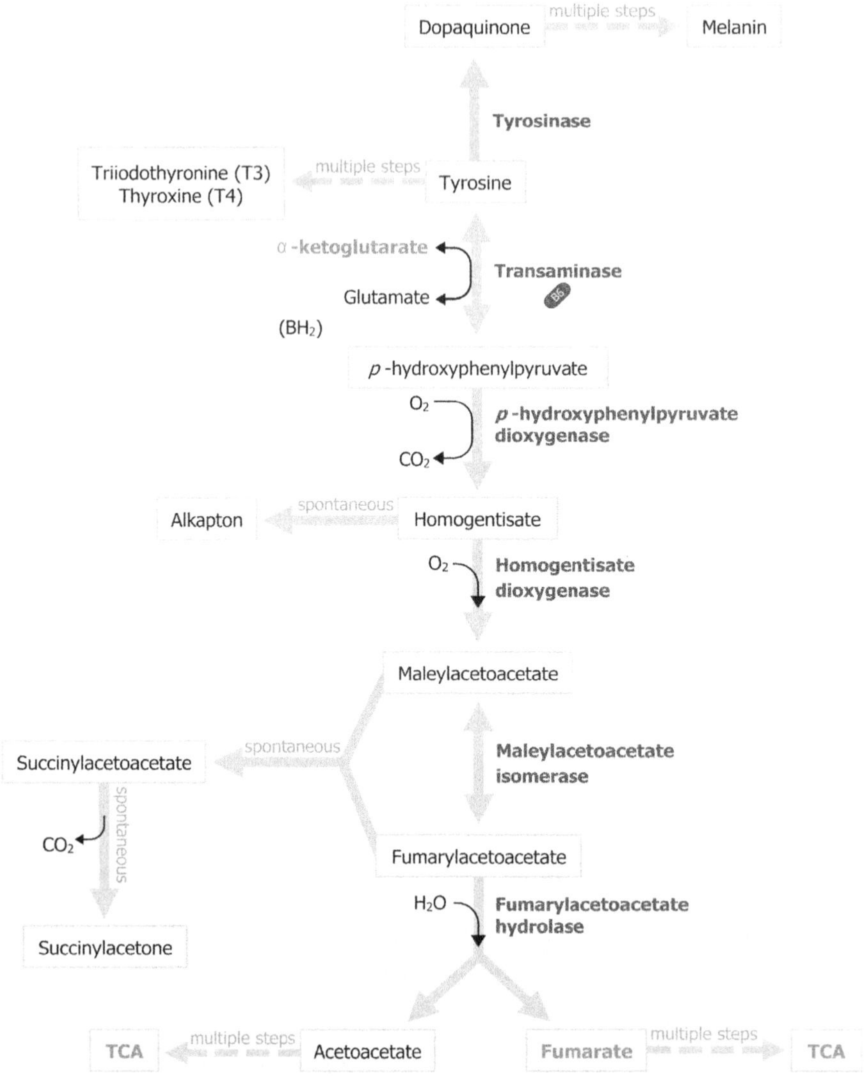

Figure 4.2: Tyrosine can be produced from phenylalanine metabolism and is required for the production of melanin and the catecholamines. Deficiencies can occur at several different locations in the pathway and result in albinism, alkaptonuria, or tyrosinemia.

Tryptophan

Tryptophan is an essential amino acid that is both ketogenic and glucogenic as it can be oxidized to produce alanine and acetyl-CoA. The ring structure can also be used to synthesize niacin, reducing the dietary requirement for this vitamin. Tryptophan metabolism to serotonin (and subsequently melatonin) requires BH_4. Deficiencies here can lead to imbalances in these neurotransmitters (figure 4.3).

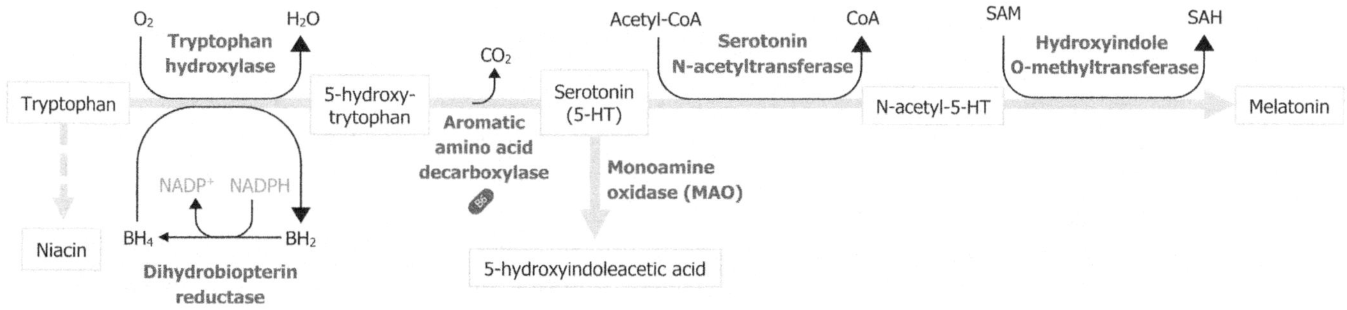

Figure 4.3: Metabolism of tryptophan to melatonin.

Glutamate

Glutamate plays many key roles in amino acid metabolism and provides substrates for GABA and glutathione synthesis (figure 4.4). Additionally, glutamate plays a role in nitrogen movement within the body. Glutamate can be deaminated by glutamate dehydrogenase to yield α-ketoglutarate. This can enter directly into the TCA cycle or be transaminated (figure 4.4). Additionally, glutamate can be used to fix or free ammonium to generate glutamine—one of the essential, nontoxic carriers of ammonia.

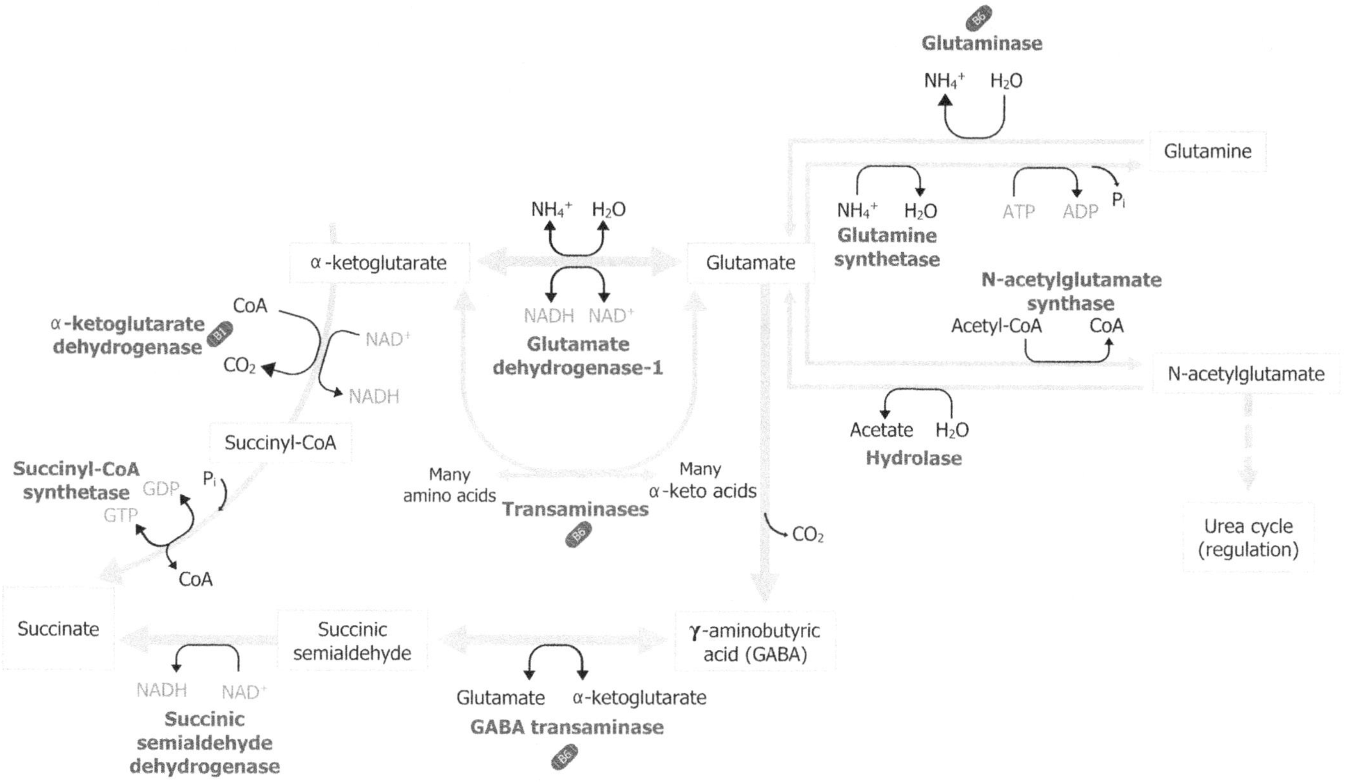

Figure 4.4: Glutamate metabolism as it interfaces with nitrogen transport and synthesis of GABA.

Isoleucine, leucine, and valine (branched-chain amino acids)

Oxidation of isoleucine, leucine, and valine, collectively described as branched-chain amino acids, occurs in all tissues and is a key fuel source for skeletal muscle. As these amino acids are approximately 25 percent of the amino acid pool, they provide both energy and available substrate to replenish the TCA cycle. The initial step in their metabolism, like all amino acids, is the transamination to generate a keto-acid. These compounds then undergo oxidative decarboxylation by a multiunit enzyme similar to the pyruvate dehydrogenase complex with similar cofactor requirements, and the remaining carbons can enter the TCA cycle.

Maple syrup urine disease

Deficiencies in the metabolism of branched-chain amino acids can result in the diagnosis of maple syrup urine disease (MSUD). With an incidence of 1 in 100,000, MSUD is rare even among the inborn errors of metabolism. However, the distinct sweet odor of the patient's urine, similar to that of maple syrup, distinguishes this condition as one of the more recognizable metabolic disorders. It is caused by deficient oxidative decarboxylation of α-keto acid metabolites of isoleucine, leucine, and valine. Affected infants can become symptomatic during the first days of life, with poor feeding, lethargy, seizures, and occasionally coma. Milder forms of MSUD may present later in life, with developmental delays and intellectual disability. Maple syrup urine disease is primarily treated by diet but also by avoiding circumstances that increase catabolism, such as high fever and dehydration. If a metabolic crisis occurs, emergency treatment in a hospital is necessary to stabilize the patient.

Methionine

Methionine is an essential amino acid with a complex metabolism of clinical importance. Its metabolism interfaces with the folate cycle, cobalamin remethylation, and the synthesis of S-adenosylmethionine (SAM). Enzymatic or cofactor deficiencies can result in elevated homocysteine levels (hyperhomocysteinemia), which can have negative impacts systemically. Methionine, required for the synthesis of SAM, can be obtained from the diet or produced from remethylation of homocysteine using vitamin B_{12}.

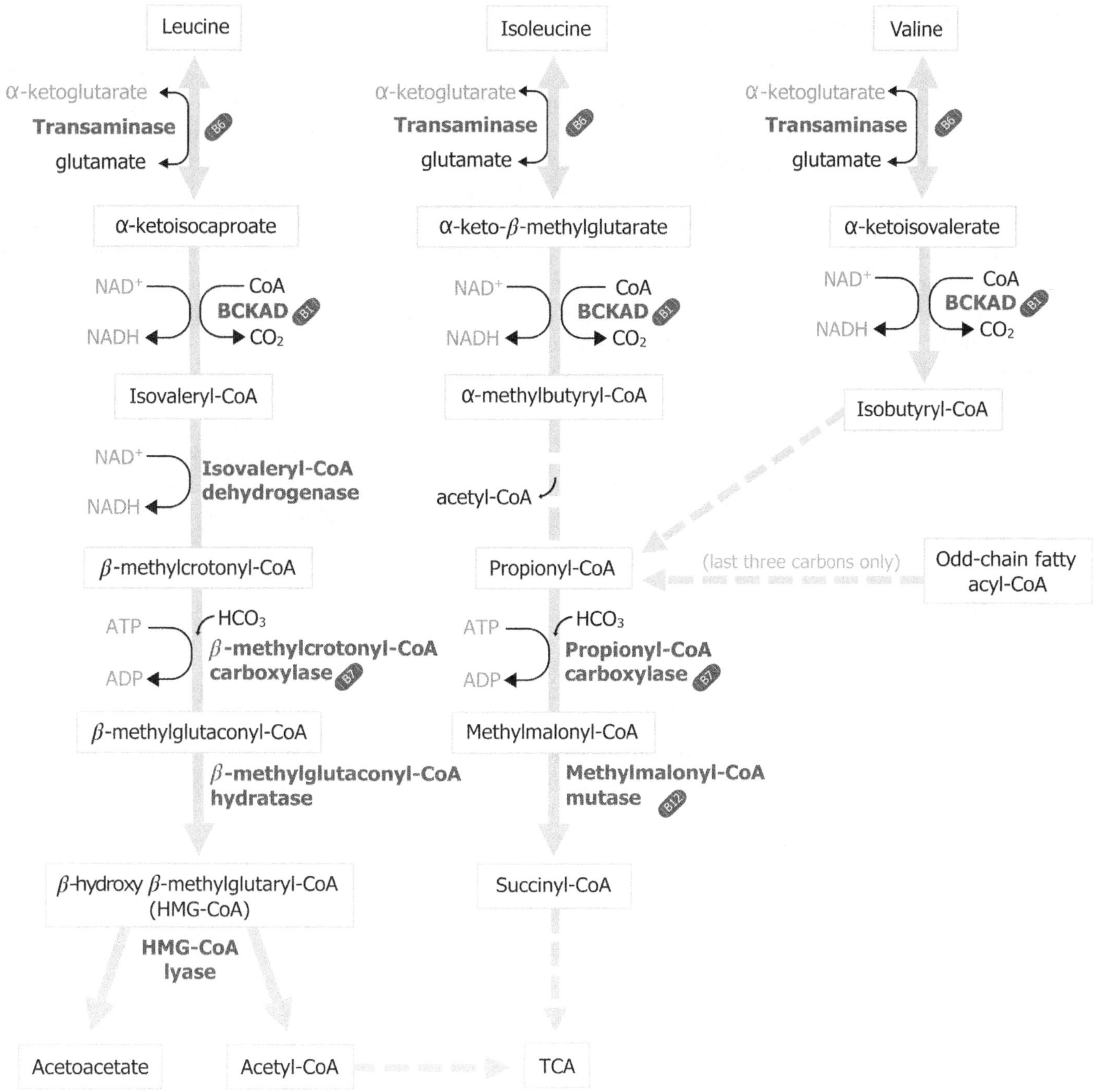

Figure 4.5: Metabolism of branched-chain amino acids. Deficiencies in branched-chain ketoacid dehydrogenase (BCKAD) can result in the presentation of maple syrup urine disease.

Initially, methionine will condense with ATP to form SAM. SAM has a charged methyl group, which can be transferred to many different acceptor molecules; this step is considered irreversible as the amount of energy released is substantial. SAM is used by many biological pathways to donate methyl groups, and it is in consistent demand. After SAM loses its methyl group, the resulting compound, S-adenosylhomocysteine (SAH), is hydrolyzed to homocysteine and adenosine. Homocysteine, generated from this reaction, can either be remethylated in a reaction using both folate and cobalamin to resynthesize methionine or can be used for the synthesis of cysteine (figure 4.6).

Remethylation of homocysteine

Homocysteine can be converted back into methionine by using both methyl-FH_4 and vitamin B_{12}. This is the only reaction in which methyl-FH_4 can donate the methyl group. In this reaction, the methyl group from FH_4 is transferred to cobalamin associated with homocysteine methyltransferase. Homocysteine receives the methyl group from this charged cobalamin cofactor, and methionine is regenerated. If homocysteine methyltransferase is defective, or if vitamin B_{12} or FH_4 levels are insufficient, homocysteine will accumulate. Elevated homocysteine levels have been linked to cardiovascular and neurologic diseases. A consequence of vitamin B_{12} deficiency is the accumulation of methyl-FH_4 and a decrease in other folate derivatives. This is known as the methyl-trap hypothesis; because of the B_{12} deficiency, most of the carbons in the FH_4 pool are trapped in the methyl-FH_4 form, which is the most stable. The carbons cannot be released from the folate because the one reaction in which they participate cannot occur due to the B_{12} deficiency. This leads to a functional folate deficiency, even though total levels of folate are normal.

A folate deficiency (whether functional or actual) leads to megaloblastic anemia caused by an inability of blood cell precursors to synthesize DNA and, therefore, to divide. This leads to large, partially replicated cells being released into the blood to attempt to replenish the cells that have died. Folate deficiencies also have been linked to an increased incidence of neural tube defects, such as spina bifida, in mothers who become pregnant while folate deficient.

Transsulfuration pathway

Further metabolism of homocysteine provides the sulfur atom for the synthesis of cysteine. In this two-step process, homocysteine first reacts with serine to form cystathionine. This is followed by cleavage of cystathionine, which yields cysteine and α-ketobutyrate. The first reaction in this sequence, catalyzed by cystathionine β-synthase, is inhibited by cysteine. Thus, methionine, via homocysteine, is not used for cysteine synthesis unless the levels of cysteine in the body are lower than required for its metabolic functions. An adequate dietary supply of cysteine, therefore, can "spare" (or reduce) the dietary requirement for methionine (figure 4.6).

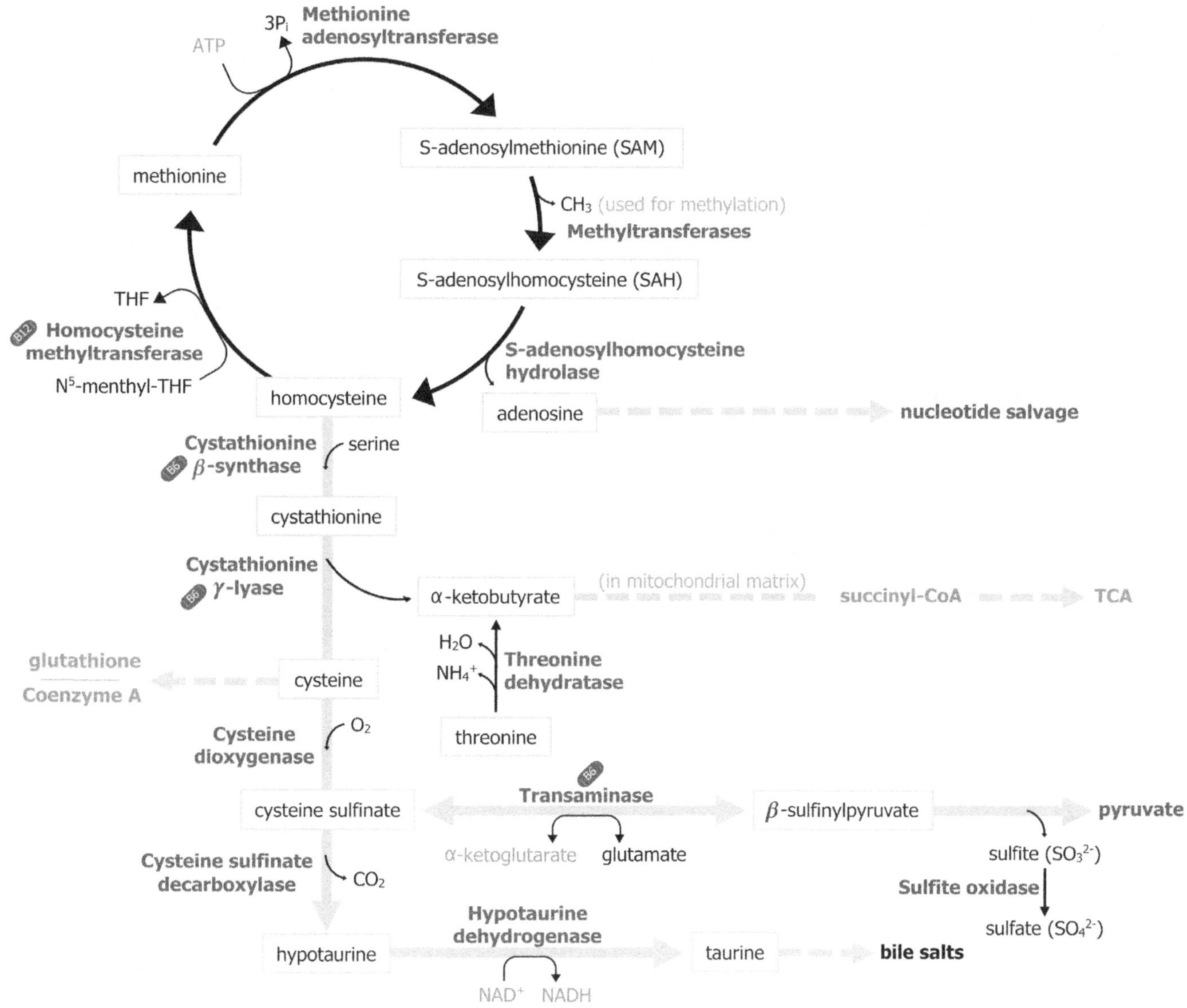

Figure 4.6: Metabolism of methionine. Remethylation and transsulfuration of homocysteine are illustrated. Cofactor or enzymatic deficiencies can result in an elevation of homocysteine.

Consequences of elevated homocysteine

Homocysteine levels can accumulate in several ways, which are related to both folic acid and vitamin B_{12} metabolism. As SAM is constantly being used as a methyl donor, this results in consistent production of SAH. Consequently, this leads to the constant production of homocysteine. The homocysteine produced can be either remethylated to methionine or condensed with serine to form cystathionine. The major pathway of homocysteine metabolism is remethylation by N 5-methyl-FH_4, which requires vitamin B_{12}. The liver also contains a second pathway in which betaine (a degradation product of choline) can donate a methyl group to homocysteine to form methionine, but this is a minor pathway. The conversion of homocysteine to cystathionine requires pyridoxal phosphate (PLP). Thus, if an individual is deficient in vitamin B_{12}, the conversion of homocysteine to methionine by the major route is inhibited. This directs homocysteine to produce cystathionine, which eventually produces cysteine. Homocysteine also accumulates in the blood if a mutation is present in the enzyme that converts N 5,N10-methylene-FH_4 to N 5-methyl-FH_4. When this occurs, the levels of N

5-methyl-FH_4 are too low to allow homocysteine to be converted to methionine. The loss of this pathway, coupled with the feedback inhibition by cysteine on cystathionine formation, also leads to elevated homocysteine levels in the blood.

A third way in which serum homocysteine levels can be elevated is by a mutated cystathionine β-synthase or a deficiency in vitamin B_6, the required cofactor for that enzyme. These defects block the ability of homocysteine to be converted to cystathionine, and the homocysteine that does accumulate cannot all be accommodated by conversion to methionine. Thus, an accumulation of homocysteine results.

References and resources

Text

Ferrier, D. R., ed. *Lippincott Illustrated Reviews: Biochemistry*, 7th ed. Philadelphia: Wolters Kluwer Health/ Lippincott Williams & Wilkins, 2017, Chapter 20: Amino Acid Degradation and Synthesis, Chapter 21: Conversion of Amino Acids to Specialized Products.

Lieberman, M., and A. Peet, eds. *Marks' Basic Medical Biochemistry: A Clinical Approach*, 5th ed. Philadelphia: Wolters Kluwer Health/Lippincott Williams & Wilkins, 2018, Chapter 37: Synthesis and Degradation of Amino Acids, Chapter 39: Tetrahydrofolate, Vitamin B12, and S-Adenosylmethionine.

Le, T., and V. Bhushan. *First Aid for the USMLE Step 1*, 29th ed. New York: McGraw Hill Education, 2018, 69, 83-85.

Figures

Figure 4.1: Metabolism of phenylalanine requires BH4 and also produces tyrosine. Grey, Kindred. "Metabolism of phenylalanine requires BH4 and also produces tyrosine. Deficiencies in cofactor or phenylalanine hydroxylase can result in phenylketonuria." 2021, https://archive.org/details/4.1_20210819. CC BY 4.0.

Figure 4.2: Tyrosine can be produced from phenylalanine metabolism and is required for the production of melanin and catecholamines. Grey, Kindred. "Tyrosine can be produced from phenylalanine metabolism and is required for the production of melanin and the catecholamines. Deficiencies can occur at several different locations in the pathway and result in albinism, alkaptonuria or tyrosinemia." 2021, https://archive.org/details/4.2_20210819. CC BY 4.0.

Figure 4.3: Metabolism of tryptophan to melatonin. Grey, Kindred. "Metabolism of Tryptophan to Melatonin." 2021, https://archive.org/details/4.3_20210819. CC BY 4.0.

Figure 4.4: Glutamate metabolism as it interfaces with nitrogen transport and synthesis of GABA. Grey, Kindred. "Glutamate metabolism as it interfaces with nitrogen transport and synthesis of GABA." 2021, https://archive.org/details/4.4_20210819. CC BY 4.0.

Figure 4.5: Metabolism of branched-chain amino acids. Grey, Kindred. "Metabolism of branched chain amino acids. Deficiencies in BCKAD can result in the presentation of Maple Syrup Urine Disease." 2021, https://archive.org/details/4.5_20210819. CC BY 4.0.

Figure 4.6: Metabolism of methionine. Grey, Kindred. “Metabolism of methionine. Remethylation and transsulfuration of homocysteine are illustrated. Cofactor or enzymatic deficiencies can result in an elevation of homocysteine.” 2021, https://archive.org/details/4.6_20210819. CC BY 4.0.

Made in the USA
Monee, IL
18 September 2022

14211535R00031